THE RULE BOOK AND USER GUIDE FOR HEALTHY LIVING

Common Sense For Black Folks Who Are Sick And Tired Of Being Sick And Tired

Nana Kwaku Opare, MD, MPH, CA

Opare Publishing, LLC
Atlanta, GA

First Edition
ISBN: 978-0-9850654-0-9
Opare Publishing, LLC
Atlanta, GA USA
www.opare.net

Rear cover photo, cover and book design by Ama T. Opare.

A healer needs to see beyond the present and tomorrow. He needs to see years and decades ahead. Because healers work for results so firm they may not be wholly visible till centuries have flowed into millennia. — Ayi Kwei Armah

This Book Is Dedicated To My Patients.

May You Heal And Be Healthy

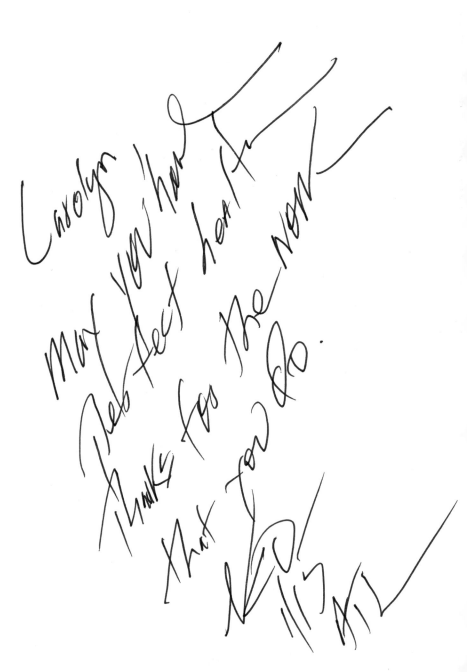

Disclaimer

This work is not to be construed as any specific medical advice. The very nature of each human life makes general advice not possible or appropriate. Please, before and during any changes you make in an attempt to heal yourself or to let anyone else try to heal you, think through the wisdom of those changes. Neither Opare Integrative Health Care, Opare Publishing, nor I will or can take responsibility for the consequences of anything you do or do not do because you read something in this book. While you may learn something herein that may help you become healthier, the information in this book is not designed to help you or anyone else treat disease.

Acknowledgements

Without the commitment toward me and the instillation in me of the value of education by my parents Marjorie B. Stepto and Herman P. Stepto (who were both first generation college and graduate school graduates), and their belief in me, I could not have navigated the minefield of the educational system.

This work could not have been completed without the love, encouragement and support of my wife and partner, Ama Thandiwe Opare, who not only is the chief executive officer, educational director and chef at Opare Integrative Health Care, but is also my best friend and biggest fan. I love you, Ama.

Thanks to Kweli Tutashinda, DC, whose talk I attended at the 2000 ASCAC regional conference in Oakland, Calif., for giving me the initial inspiration to develop this rule book.

Without the inspiration of the Egungun and the Loa, I could not have completed this work. Ashe.

Mwalimu Baruti and Marimba Ani have personally inspired me by their consistent and clear fulfillment of their Ori.

Medase Baruti for reading an early draft of this work and telling me that we have a book here. Medase Yaa Baruti for the proverbs.

Thanks to Yemi Toure, who not only edited the manuscript but who also taught my first course in mass media at Pitzer College in the 1970s. That course was instrumental in showing me that not all that we see and hear is true. I have made all the final edits and revisions and as such take responsibility for any errors and/or omissions in the text.

Table of Contents

The Rule Book And User Guide For Healthy Living
Common Sense For Black Folks
Who Are Sick And Tired Of Being Sick And Tired

Foreword

We as Afrikan* people have always understood and experienced ourselves holistically.

*We spell Afrika with a "k" because it is spelled that way in Kiswahili, the most widely spoken Black language in the world. By doing this, we are saying that "the Afrikan way" of doing things is a good way.

We have never made any meaningful distinctions between our spiritual, psychological and physical manifestations because they are intimately, inextricably, irrefutably interconnected. To us, the seen and unseen are concretely and intuitively recognized as one energized, creative, indivisible, vital force.

The idea that Afrikans see themselves as being one with the Universe is unfathomable to the yurugu[1] mind, determined to "scientifically" fragment and polarize everything in the Universe. Our unity with the Universe is something that we positively know in the timeless, infinite depths of our consciousness, a collective consciousness that rises from our spirit to enlighten our mind and purposefully animate our physical presence. It is a consciousness that could only be created out of this oneness.

For Afrikans, this holistic interpretation of reality naturally instructs and orders the healing process. Our true physicians have never attended to physical symptoms isolated from their mental and spiritual components. We know that one aspect of being cannot be damaged without the others being also damaged and, therefore, there is no healing one without healing the others. The patient is physical, mental and spiritual, as well as familial and communal. When we become imbalanced, there is no remedying of one aspect of our being without attending to related causal or affected imbalances in the others. Healing the body requires a concomitant healing of the mind and spirit. Healing the mind requires a concomitant healing of the body and spirit. And healing the spirit requires a concomitant healing of the body and mind. The three are inextricably intertwined.

Of course being who we originally are, a people forged in the love of community, what ails us is never separated from the community of individuals of whom we are inseparable. It is an extended family, spiritually, physically and mentally tied. Therefore, the healing of the patient's family/community is equally critical to healing the patient's mind, body and spirit.

It is from this fundamental, holistic-oriented Afrikan truth that Nana Kwaku Opare works and teaches. As a seasoned physician, a healer in the Afrikan tradition, Nana knows what we need to heal because he speaks through the medical mind of our ancestors. And, because of this grounding and orientation, in this book he offers sound guidelines for us to recover our health within an Afrikan center.

It should be noted that seldom do we find a healing talent and Afrikan mind in the same person. Even rarer is such an individual who is willing to make the time to explain to a community so unhealthily distanced from our origins how we must approach living if we are to return to our prime physical, mental, spiritual and communal existence. Nana Kwaku Opare is one such healer. Without doubt, he embodies this ancestral truth, and this book clearly reflects his vision, mission and passion for helping to rebuild a whole Afrikan people.

Mwalimu Baruti

Baruti is a scholar, educator and author of many books about Afrikan people.

Author's Foreword

Before healing others, heal yourself. — Gambian

In my first year of high school, I knew I wanted to be either an architect or a physician. A mediocre grade in a drafting class and the top grade in a biology class sealed my fate.

My original given name was Steven, and I was born into the Stepto family of Chicago. The adults in my family have been for generations mostly teachers and civic employees. My father's brother, Robert Stepto, was an influential physician who achieved many honors, including the chair of several academic and clinical departments of Ob/Gyn, chair of the Board of Health of the City of Chicago, and president of the International College of Surgeons. Uncle Bob's success showed me that becoming a physician was something I could and was possibly born to do. The only child of my educator parents (my father remarried and had my sister Kelley while I was in high school), I grew up on the South Side of Chicago in the Chatham and Hyde Park neighborhoods. My childhood and youth were privileged and free of serious trauma.

I was a peculiar and wild child, but managed to stay out of trouble and graduate from high school with good enough grades to get me into college.

My initial motivation was to be successful in life and to be like Uncle Bob. Even though that is a great goal for any youth, it was not enough for me. I realized, perhaps in my nascent Afrikan consciousness, that I wanted to help as many people as I possibly could, as much as I possibly could, as a physician. I felt an early calling to help our people heal.

Only too eager to escape the Chicago winters, I matriculated at Pitzer College in Claremont, Calif., majoring in biology. While there, my political awakening occurred. (My cultural awakening would have to wait more than 20 years.) I became aware of the nature of race and class in our society. I realized that to help as many people as possible to heal would require a public health approach. It became abundantly obvious that diet was the key factor in the improvement or deterioration of good health.

Transferring to the University of California at Berkeley, I changed my major to Food, Nutrition and Dietetics. My undergraduate education was rigorous and not a lot of fun. I had more courses in chemistry than any subject other than my major. I was blessed to assist in the labs of two of the most famous and respected academics in nutrition, George Briggs, Ph.D., and Doris Calloway, Ph.D. Even though in the 1970s the data showed veganism to be the healthiest diet, the concept was never bandied about in Morgan Hall, the home of the Department of Nutrition at Cal. We were taught we needed cooked animal protein and dairy to be healthy and vital. My own independent research, my growing wisdom and my common sense later proved that to be inaccurate.

Graduating from Cal with my bachelor of science in food, nutrition and dietetics, I matriculated in the M.D./M.P.H. program at UCSF, finishing my dual degree program in the mid-1980s. I completed my internship at Highland Hospital-Alameda County Medical Center in Oakland, Calif.

Medical school and internship were spiritually difficult for me. They were degrading to my sense of rightness and order. I saw the futility and inhumanity of what passes as medicine in our society. I saw the depersonalization and objectification of patients, which the student doctor is conditioned to do in the name of "objectivity."

This objectification was seriously flawed, and when it came to poor, Black or other patients of color, was absent. I came to see the closed-minded and elitist nature of allopathic (standard Western) medicine. I also experienced the futility and ineffectiveness of what passes as modern medicine. I saw hundreds of thousands of dollars spent ushering terminal patients (draining into the coffers of the hospitals, drug and medical equipment companies and the doctors who worked for them whatever remaining wealth they had) painfully as slowly as possible, to their graves. Patients whose families were given false hope, reduced to artificially maintained life forms with virtually zero chance of returning to any semblance of normal existence. I have witnessed what should have been labeled atrocities causing untold suffering inflicted on patients in the quest to "preserve life at all costs." This ordeal occasionally helped the patient get better and function, but always cost the patient their dignity and bank account, and almost always failed to restore true health.

Patients are sliced and diced with a resulting mere semblance of normalcy, propped up by dependency on chemicals that would, with alarming frequency, ultimately poison and kill them. I saw people reduced from human beings into their clinical diagnosis — stripped of their dignity and humanity. I saw a complete lack of attention to prevention and such simple basics as exercise, fresh air, proper food and water. I saw a complete absence of spirit in the practice of allopathic medicine. I experienced a systematic pattern of white supremacy/racism, and the lie of cultural Darwinism[2] infused deeply and inextricably in every facet of the medical establishment.

I saw a pervasive lack of intellectual honesty in physicians who refused to acknowledge any alternatives to the orthodoxy that was originally installed by those in power. These chiefs of medicine in hospitals and medical schools often were holding their positions for life. Their pronouncements and edicts as to what was true or false concerning the human organism were, I later discovered, more often than not based on a thirst for power than for truth. Truth be damned. The quest for grants and prestige trumped what was truly best for the patient and their families.

My professional-level training in nutrition and dietetics found no utility in medical school. I often heard chiefs of departments pronounce that it does not matter what the patient ate. But this was something I knew from studying at Berkeley to be false. This ignorance, which I could only conclude was willful, was made painfully obvious because out of the thousands of hours of lectures I attended, only a few hours were devoted to nutrition. And these few were so basic and non-specific that I could have given them myself extemporaneously. Any lectures in nutrition were unusual. Only one in four

U.S. medical schools at that time, and even today, offer any lectures in nutrition.[3] The famous adage known to have been originated by Imhotep and later appropriated by Hippocrates, "Let food be thy medicine and medicine be thy food," was ignored.

... from UCSF, we were led in reciting ... cal oath instead. I alone in my class ... ecite this oath, knowing it to be a lie ... . I vowed instead to do my part to ... as it helps. Since then, I have found ... onely as my graduation was. I have ... ctors willing or able to question the ... a form of medicine that arrogantly ... fails to toe the line of the medical ... up an obscene 17.4 percent of our ... per year. Complications brought on by ... eading cause of death in the United ... states.

... t the design of my Egungun that UCSF ... ental medicine collection in the library. ... my path. Oddly enough, this extensive ... the medical school curriculum. There ... ass of a proposed mechanism for how ... was about it. Herbal medicine was not ... in medical school I found in the school ... to become my primary textbook of ... se Acupuncture" is a fascinating and ... study this ancient and powerful healing

... nto a residency program in my chosen, ... gency medicine, I enrolled in the San ... and Oriental Medicine. SFCAOM was one ... riental medicine in the 1980s. I completed ... arded the right to use the CA designation.

Since becoming board certified in 1987, I have been active in the field of traditional Chinese medicine, serving on the faculty at Meiji College of Oriental Medicine and the American College of Traditional Chinese Medicine. I served as consultant to the National Commission for the Certification of Acupuncture and Oriental Medicine. I helped write the board examinations used to license acupuncturists throughout the country. Even though I enjoyed my appointments, it became clear to me that a career in TCM alone was not my path.

In 1992 I was fortunate to meet a physical therapist who recommended a series of continuing education courses in osteopathic manual medicine, offered by the Michigan State College of Osteopathic Medicine. I was in heaven when I found my gift for hands-on manipulative medicine. There is nothing more satisfying to me than laying my hands on patients and seeing the smile on their faces as they feel better and are relieved of their back or neck pain. I have continued to complete almost the entire curriculum of hands-on courses to refine my craft over the past 20 years. I was blessed to study (among the other outstanding faculty at Michigan State) with Philip Greenman, DO, and with my mentor in acupuncture, the late Dr. Andrew Tseng. They were not only the two best teachers of medicine I have ever had, but also the best clinicians. To this very day when I perform an osteopathic manipulation, I envision Dr. Greenman's hands, and when I perform acupuncture, I envision Dr. Tseng's.

I am often asked how I came to be named Nana Kwaku Opare and am I an enstooled Akan priest? I am not enstooled however during my trip to Ghana in 1996, I was given my spiritual name in ceremony at the Akonedi Shrine, after and in honor of the late Okomfohemma Nana Akua Oparebea, high priestess of the Akonedi Shrine at Larteh, Ghana.[6] It was years later I legally changed my name to Opare.

I continued to practice both TCM and allopathic emergency medicine (incorporating osteopathic manual therapy into my allopathic practice) and later urgent care and occupational medicine separately. I opened my own private practice in integrating TCM, allopathic medicine and nutritional medicine in Oakland, Calif., in 2004. Over the past several years I have refined my clinical technique, formulating the Opare Method ™.

Through my experience and through divination, I have come to understand that my gifts for healing and teaching were given to me to help Afrikan people. This is what brought me to Atlanta.

Parallel to my medical training was a change in my own diet. I began my transition into veganism while in college in the 1970s. I severely cut back on all flesh and eggs. Given my good health, it was hard to consider a serving of fish once or twice a month to be hazardous. I came to the conclusion that no amount of animal products is safe. So I gave up fish.

I was already vegan when the "mad cow" disease scare surfaced, and it became clear it could be transmitted through all animal products. It has been a no-brainer to stay on my path since.

I have been blessed with good health my entire life. As such, I have been able to adjust my diet to prevent illness. With the exception of a pretty severe allergic rhinitis that went away when I quit dairy, I have been well.

It took me the better part of two decades to accept a total vegan lifestyle. Unfortunately, today's risks of continued animal product consumption are so severe, I cannot recommend a slow transition to veganism for even the healthiest people today. I advise all who will listen that if they want to restore or protect their health, a rapid and permanent transition to veganism is an essential first step.

I have been blessed with the privilege of watching people change their lives through changing how they eat. My experience has led me to understand that you cannot eat your way to health, but you can eat your way to the grave. Changing your diet is an essential part of claiming your perfect health. However, eating in alignment with your body's natural constitution is only one of many things you must do if you want to cooperate with your God-given gift of perfect health.

This book has been a while coming and while the ideas all are there, the reader may want for more explanation and detail in defense of my ideas. I came to the conclusion that the time to get this work out was now. As such there may be omissions or errors that if left longer in gestation would have matured out of this text.

May this book help you on your path.

NKO

Why Yet Another Book On Health?

Africa is our center of gravity, our cultural and spiritual mother and father, our beating heart, no matter where we live on the face of this Earth. — John Henrik Clarke

Most books I have picked up about health or nutrition have not only been too thick but too hard to comprehend. If there are too many words that the average person has to use a dictionary to understand, then the book is going to do more to confuse than to make things clear.

More information does not equal more understanding. If I write a book, what good is it if it doesn't help readers to *understand* the topic? Unless my true goal is to lead them to further confusion to keep them from making the right decisions that might ultimately lead them to not need my services or goods anymore.

Many if not most authors, for the purposes of financial gain and/or self-aggrandizement, are trying to impress readers and their colleagues about how much of an expert they are. They are trying to convince readers that they are clever, more so than the person who wrote the last book on the topic. They want readers to believe that the authors are naturally brilliant and gifted, and/or through years of study and hard-fought experience, are special. They want readers to believe they know all the "right" / "famous" / "important" people in the field who are also special, and who have anointed them with the knowledge that will change the readers' lives. They want you to believe they are smarter than you, and that is why you must read their book in order to reveal "the secret."

I'm going to try not to do any of this. Instead I will try to put what I know as plainly as I can. I am going to try to convince you that you are smarter than me and anyone else — at least when it comes to your own health and if you clear all the clutter from the fifty-eleven sources of information you have in front of you, you will discover the plain truth — you already have everything you need to heal anything — in you right now.

If you are able to access that God-given wisdom of your own common sense and become aware of the messages you are constantly being given from the Divine; if you are able to think things through for yourself, and quit relying on experts to tell you what is in front of your face, you are on your way to perfect health. If you then learn to make thorough and careful observation of your own bodily sensations and intuitions, you will learn what does and doesn't make sense for you and your family on how to get or stay healthy. This book is about helping you do just that.

I hope by making what I have to say as plain and simple as possible, able to stand on its own logic, I can help you in your process of self-discovery/healing. Although I will include references, it is my intention that this book does not rely on previously published materials to prove its points. If my points cannot be verified by your own common sense, I have failed.

This is a book for Afrikan people. It is for us, by us. There are plenty of works by Europeans and those who think as they do, written for Europeans and those who live as they do. This one is for Afrikans. It is about our personal and our collective health. What goes into creating a healthy life will vary depending on where you come from and the history of your family. Afrikan people have unique and distinct cultural characteristics and needs that people of European or Asian or other extractions do not share. I hope to shed light on this herein.

I don't pretend that I have the final answer to how to get and stay healthy. In fact, I don't claim to have any knowledge that is unique or that I came to through divine inspiration. I do not pretend that there is something new or different to say — there isn't. It has all been said or written about before. Your grandmother, the old woman down the street, the village diviner, Imhotep, Queen Afua, Muata Ashby, Laila Afrika, Dick Gregory and others said it. You have known it throughout your entire life — if you chose to heed the knowledge within. What I am writing you here is about instinct and its human corollary, intuition, and it is also about divine inspiration and ancestral guidance.

What is my gift? I hope to bring a way of looking at health that makes it less confusing, less frightening or daunting a task, more accessible, and most importantly, less susceptible to the vast and overwhelming health propaganda flooding the mass media that keeps us paralyzed, stuck doing the same old things we have always done; mindlessly going through our days with the same old bad habits; continuing to live the same unhealthy addictive patterns of behavior that drive the economy and continue to perpetuate our mental and economic enslavement. These are the same behaviors that continue to fill the coffers of the fast-food, drug, tobacco and medical industries.

I hope that this work may help the reader to go back to that which once served all living beings. That is using your own personal experience, that of your parents and elders around you and your divine gift of intuition to make life decisions. I encourage you to make up your own mind and trust your age-old customs and traditions; learn from your mistakes and institute changes in your life. I want to make it plain, to distill or better yet simplify sometimes complex information and make it available to the average person. I hope that through reading this you are more able to heed your own inner wisdom, to use your own common sense, to come to first trust yourself and your own ability to discern what is good for you and your loved ones.

This work is about common sense. It is about mental, physical, emotional and spiritual health. It is about coming to understand the mass mental disease we have been afflicted with that manifests in collective and individual addictive dysfunctional patterns of living and thinking. It is about recovering from this yurugu illness. It is about recovering from self-destructive behavior that perpetuates our mental enslavement and our illnesses for the "profit" of a few.

This book is about finally learning to trust your own ability to think through things for yourself. It is about shedding the naiveté that most people possess about getting and staying well. It is about understanding that most of what we have been told, and most of what is customary around our health, is erroneous and counterproductive to getting healthy and staying healthy.

Sadly, even those who should be the most trusted sources of information, our parents, are often wrong. After generations of misinformation and corporate propaganda, most of what has even been passed down to us is not helpful for staying or getting well. This work is about you learning to judge health information by using your common sense. If something makes sense when you critically think about it, it is more than likely true. If something does not make sense, it is more than likely false.

"Any effort to understand the problems of disease that refuses to see the phenomena of disease in the light of cause and effect is doomed to disappointment. What horrid superstition, what blinding prejudice, what unpalliated stupidity is that which cannot understand the simple doctrine that diseases are remediable by (and only by) removing their causes! What is there so difficult to understand about the simple principle that in order to be saved from the effects of a practice, it is necessary to discontinue the practice? How absurd to think that the practice can be continued and poisons administered to erase or prevent its effects! The production of effects can be ended only by removing the causes that are producing them. The medical man acts as though he believes that effects can be erased and their production ended without the necessity of removing their causes."

(Herbert M. Shelton, "Natural Hygiene — Man's Pristine Way Of Life," 1968, Dr. Shelton's Health School, San Antonio, Texas.)

Also, this book reflects my as-of-yet-incomplete understanding of Afrikan culture and spirituality. My understanding of health and healing are a work in progress. Please excuse any ambiguity or confusion. I will make corrections and additions in future editions of this work and in other texts.

Despite the title in my name, I am not enstooled or an akomfo.[7] I am not a priest of any type. I am a physician. I have come to see the inseparable nature of spiritual and physical health. I have found that spiritual illness is more than anything else at the root of our health problems as Afrikan people. In order to heal ourselves, we must heal the spirit. In ancient times before the Maafa,[8] the root of all healing was done through the spirit world.

If we as modern Afrikan doctors fail to realize this, we will fail to heal our people.

Have You Got Your Health Assurance Card?

Health has no price. — Swahili

In the United States, health is often the hot topic in national discussion and debate. The majority of the discussion is around health insurance. Who has it? Who doesn't? Is it a right or is it a privilege? Who should pay for it? Much less discussion is around what does it pay for and what are you really insuring?

The fear of getting sick, suffering and perishing from some horrible illness is real and increasing. For good reason, rates of serious chronic illnesses like diabetes and cancer are rising rapidly. The prospect of having to pay for these illnesses is daunting. The fear of not being able to afford medical care when we do get sick is also rising. That fear is real. Medical care costs are spiraling out of control. In 2009, 17.4 percent of the U.S. GDP (gross domestic product) went to the medical industry. This portion has been steadily rising. The country with the next largest bite is The Netherlands 12.0 percent.[9] Hospitalization can cost more than $10,000 per day. Medications can cost hundreds and even thousands of dollars per month. Physician bills, dental bills, medical equipment bills, rehabilitation and physical therapy bills, dialysis and so on are beyond the cost of the majority of the population. Only the wealthy can imagine ever paying these bills out of pocket. No surprise our preoccupation on health care insurance.

More and more people are going bankrupt as a result of medical bills. A 2007 Harvard study found sixty-two percent of bankruptcies are due to medical bills. This percentage has been climbing precipitously since 2001. This is sad enough in and of itself. Even sadder is that in three-quarters of these medical bankruptcies, the person had health insurance.[10] In other words, these folks thought they did everything right. They played by the rules. They held down that good job that gave them health insurance that would protect them and their family financially in case of illness — and they still went broke. This is a travesty and a betrayal of the system we have been sold to believe is the "best in the world."

There is little evidence to suggest that the U.S. system of medical care results in healthier people.[11] But what is clear is that it results in poorer people. You don't just have medical bills when you get sick — you eventually stop having income. For most of us, after a couple of weeks at best, it is no work no pay. Get sick — get broke!

Think about it. What is health insurance anyway? We are paying some company our money and are betting them that we are going to get sick and we hope we lose and then they get to keep our money. They are also betting us our money that we don't get sick and then they get to keep our money. Sounds like a losing proposition for everyone except the insurance companies. More and more doctors are quitting, getting out of the medical business. The No. 1 reason doctors cite when they quit is outside influence and bureaucracy[12] (read that as health insurance companies) are making it harder and harder for them to do their job and make a good living.

Aside from all this, the "health insurance" our job provides us does nothing to keep us healthy. The health insurance product benefits us only when we get sick. And who wants to get sick?

So do we actually want to be healthy? Not as evidenced by our behavior. The risk factors for most illnesses have been known for decades. Public health statistics have shown a rise in diseases that have a clear and preventable cause and a drop in diseases that are due to causes beyond our control. Yet the behaviors that lead to these illnesses persist and in fact are accelerating. It should come as no surprise that the population as a whole is ignorant of the causes of (the almost entirely preventable) major killers and disablers of citizens of the industrialized world and now increasingly the developing world. Follow the money. Who stands to profit if merely changing our behavior can keep us from getting sick? You can bet it isn't Eli Lilly, McDonald's, Sutter Health or even Aetna.

We have become a country of reckless drivers when it comes to our health. No wonder our insurance premiums keep rising. What is worse is that we have been sold the idea that disease is something that just happens to us. Is it the luck of the draw, or is it a result of bad genes? Is it a result of poisons in the environment we have no control over? Or is it virulent insidious microbes poised to infect us? None of this is something we can effectively control. So why bother trying. Just keep on doing what you have been doing. There is no need to take care if taking care will make no difference.

We have been sold this idea that when we "crash" or break down our bodies, we can just go to the human body shop (hospital or clinic) and see our human body mechanic (doctor or other health practitioner) and after pulling out our insurance card, they will fix us back as good as new or at least get us back on the road again. We don't have to pull cash out of our pockets. We are comforted in the knowledge that because we have insurance we can go along our merry way smoking, drinking, and eating "food-like substances" and get away scot-free.

Remember the age-old adage — an ounce of prevention is worth a pound of cure. The funny thing is that most of us have forgotten this. The even funnier thing is that most of us believe that no matter what we do as we age, we will become sick and debilitated. We don't believe that we can feel great and be vibrant and productive well into our later years. And why should we believe otherwise? We see very few examples of those who do. We dismiss them as freaks of nature and fall back into our life-destroying habits.

We are confused by the smorgasbord of health misinformation out there — almost all of which is paid for by those who seek to capitalize on our illness or at least our fear of it. It is very profitable and good for business if people do not think they can do anything to keep themselves well. Or that only those who are weird zealots and extremists could possibly do that which would keep themselves well. So we go along our merry way committing slow suicide and dooming a large portion of ourselves and our heirs to insolvency. All the while we believe we are living the American dream when we are (if we take a sober look at it) slowly dying the American nightmare of disease, disability, suffering, insolvency and death itself.

Affirmation: I will bet my money and my life on my good health, and hope I win. I invest in those things that have been proven to promote health and expect to reap dividends as I age. I choose to believe that I can feel good and be healthy if I take proper care of myself. I choose to believe that debilitation and illnesses are not the inevitable result of aging. I choose to believe that my health, like a good car, if I assiduously maintain it, will run great and look great as long as I choose to own it or live. I choose not to spend my money on the expense of health insurance.[13] I chose to invest my money in health assurance. I choose to do that which will keep my body vehicle running well and my money in my bank account, not in some mega insurance company. I choose to make my decisions on how I live my life on what is prudent, wise and safe for my health, and not on what is decadent, capricious and reckless. I choose to eat wisely, exercise wisely and not poison myself with drugs, tobacco, alcohol or coffee. I enjoy feeling good and vital and not having to depend on pills or the hope that when I inevitably get sick, I don't go broke. I choose, when I die, to leave my money to my heirs and not the hospital and drug industry. I choose to spend my money on good, clean, organic food; yoga and tai chi classes, and therapy and spiritual work that will pay me lifelong dividends in feeling better while I am alive. I bet my money on staying healthy and I am confident I will win!

The Sacred Nature Of Being

The most difficult thing to get people to do is to accept the obvious. — Dick Gregory

All of us know deep down inside what it takes to be healthy and whole. We have it coded into our DNA. It is in our ancestral memory. It is our instinct. Living in harmony with the planet is, as it is for all beings, our birthright and our sacred duty.

But some people are incomplete beings, born without that drive or desire or need to harmonize. These damaged souls have a desire to dominate and control other people and the planet. They see the world as something that is to be taken and used.[14]

This way of being in the world ultimately leads them to neglecting their gifts. This way of interacting leaves these flawed souls seeing health and life itself as only a mechanistic, chemical reaction. This view of life is desacralized,[15] void of spirit and thus not subject to higher control, responsibility or ethical duty. It leads to a "scientific" doctrine that defines humans as mere "things" that can be altered for profit.

That cultural/social/psychological flaw is yurugu.[16] Yurugu spreads like a virus and has nearly infected the whole of humanity. It appears that only small pockets of humanity have avoided infection. Ultimately, we as part of the biomass of this planet and all living things are in dire danger of succumbing to it. Perhaps this is part of the natural order of things — for life here to end this way. (I pray this is not the case and that we are now in the maximum depth of Isfet[17] and are coming out of it into khephra.)[18]

We as Afrikan people must come to see that this is not our way. We must remind ourselves that all is sacred, that our way is to understand and function in the world with respect and reverence for what God has created. We must return to our way of harmonizing with our environment and all that is in it. This way is fundamental to our health as it is for all species.

Not~So~Common Sense

Throughout this work you will find catchy phrases to take with you on your daily travels and to help you wade through the muck of misinformation and sales propaganda masquerading as health information. If these phrases prove over time to be wise, they may become proverbs. Proverbs help us preserve and transmit wisdom to our youth. They remind us how to act in a proper way.

If You Have Been Given Something Of Value, Show Your Appreciation And Take Care Of It

Why is it most of us take better care of our cars than we do our health? Having "health" insurance is no more taking care of your health than having auto insurance is taking care of your car. You get one body in this life. Why abuse or neglect it and then assume because you have insurance you will get fixed right up? That's like driving recklessly and never changing your oil, cleaning the car or tuning it and expecting it to serve you well. That doesn't happen with your car or your body. Have health insurance for the same reason you have auto insurance. Live carefully and take care of your body, mind and spirit and if by chance you crash, you may be able to afford to get it fixed. But just like a fixed-up car, a fixed-up body is never quite the same.

If We Took Care Of Our Money Like We Do Our Health, We Would Be Flat Broke

It is your responsibility to take care of your health. It is spiritual law that what you pay your attention to is what you give energy to.

Health Is Our Only True Wealth

Each of us has a gift we were given when we were born; it is our duty to use that gift in service to the world. This is called being on purpose. Being on purpose means doing your best to help your family and community. You can only do this if you are healthy in body, mind and spirit.

Also, lose your health — lose your wealth. Most bankruptcies occur as a result of medical bills — and most of those are filed by people who had "health" insurance. Michael Moore documented this well in his movie "Sicko."

If You Are Tired — Rest

You don't need more tonics; you need more sleep. I often have patients who complain of fatigue. The first thing I ask them is, "Are you getting enough sleep?" More often than not the answer is no. My response is, "Let's do what we can to get you the sleep you need, and if at that point you are still feeling tired, then let's look into other options." I'll ask, "Why are you not getting enough sleep?" Frequently the answer is, "I have too much to do."

Focus on getting your life together and getting the sleep you need. Then, come back and see me if you still are tired. Sleep first, check thyroid, CBC, etc., later.

If You Are Weak — Exercise

This one is often hard for me. I tend to be lazy and like to put my face in a good movie or book. The fact is, "use it or lose it." That which we ignore or don't use will tend to go away. If you are young, it is easy to forget this and think you can always get it back. It is a lot easier and less work to stay in shape than to let yourself go, and then get back in shape. Our tendency is to prioritize other things like family and business. We will take jobs or other responsibilities and not leave time for exercise. This is folly. What are you working for? Are you working to feel bad? Are you working to build financial wealth at the expense of your only true wealth — your bodily and mental health? I always advise younger family men and women not to take a job a long way from home. Why? Because the time they spend commuting is frequently taken from the time that would have otherwise been used to take care of themselves. Take a job you can ride your bicycle to. Get to work and stay in shape at the same time.

If You Are Stiff — Stretch

It is astonishing to me how often this simple rule is forgotten. When you are tight and it is hard to move, doing routine day-to-day tasks are more difficult. Yoga is a great way to keep your body supple and flexible. Take a few minutes each morning to incorporate a few simple yoga poses such as child's pose, spinal twists, or sun salutations to start your day off right.

If You Are Hungry — Eat

The reverse of this is more important. If you ain't hungry you cain't (must not) eat. This sounds simple, but it is in fact difficult for most of us. Very few people actually know when they are truly hungry. Our desires for food are regulated by the clock — it's noon? Must be lunchtime. We mistake boredom, anger or loneliness for hunger. Learning to disengage from the "food as entertainment" or "food as drug" mentality of our culture is a big step toward putting food and eating into proper perspective.

If You Have Too Much On Your Mind — Stop Thinking

Meditate. Worrying and struggling over something rarely solves the problem. Instead it impacts our sleep, our eating and our lives. Taking time to meditate, to "let go and let God" allows us to reach deep within to a place that is difficult to find in the midst of thinking. It allows us to hear our intuition, our ancestors, and the divine spirit speaking to us. It is in these seemingly unproductive times that peace and inspiration are born.

If You Feel Full — . . .

When you eat in alignment with your body's constitution, you will naturally have regular bowel movements each day. It is a natural process to move your bowels following a meal. It is one of the ways your body flushes out toxins as well as waste products. Eat lots of fruits and veggies and drink plenty of water to keep your pipes flushing regularly.

If It's White — Don't Bite

White sugar, white flour, white salt, white potato, cocaine, white aspirin, white milk, white rice and white bread. These processed items are de-natured, adulterated, addictive, devoid of nutrients, unnatural and unnecessary. White stuff is just bad for you, period. Avoid it; don't put it in your mouth.

Nobody Can Heal You But You

This is one of the most important concepts I teach. All healing occurs in only one place. That is inside of you. It is your bodily processes that effect the healing. Even if you are surgical post-op and you had the best surgeon in the world, it is you and God who do the healing. If your body/mind/spirit/soul are not ready to heal, then there is nothing anybody else can do to help. If your body/mind/spirit/soul are ready to heal, God will see to it you do.

If It Ain't Broke — Don't Fix It

Many people come to my office to get "maintenance treatments." This is especially true with chiropractic care. But I have found that treatment is not maintenance — it is repair. Take proper care of your body. Even if you have mild symptoms, this means you have not been taking care of yourself properly — you need to redouble your maintenance. Unlike your car, maintenance is something you can do for yourself. Go in for repairs (treatments) only if you are broken.

Five Adages For Healthy Living

The doctor cannot drink the medicine for the patient. — Tshi

False belief: we must in the course of life become ill. When we do, we must submit to our physicians and do what they say to get better. My doctor always knows what's best for me.

Remember #1 - Forget The Rest.

#1 Don't Get Sick

#2 If You Do Get Sick, Don't Go See Anyone

#3 If You Go See Someone, Don't Go See An M.D.

#4 If You Go See An M.D., Don't Go See A Surgeon

#5 If You Go See A Surgeon, Don't Go See One At A Teaching Hospital

#1 Don't Get Sick

This is the most important part of good health. The truth is that it is the hardest part as well. How can anyone control whether they get sick or not?

Most illnesses don't come from chance or bad luck or bad genes. Most illnesses and diseases (and some metaphysicians would even include injuries) come about because of failure to properly care for ourselves. A very small percentage are the result of karmic debt. Karma cannot be escaped and the consequences of bad and good karma will inescapably affect our lives. Bad karma can result in illness. The vast majority of illnesses result from failing to follow the Rule Book and User Guide agreed to by us and installed in our subconscious at birth.[19] The natural response to disease or dis-ease is to first identify and remove the cause, because our body has built-in natural mechanisms for restoring balance. We deep inside know what we did or failed to do to get sick. We also have the power to change those things and heal.

Paradoxically, sometimes what appears as illness is in fact a sign of proper functioning of the human organism. We are living in a toxic society both mentally and physically. We will tend to accumulate those toxins in our bodies and minds. In their wisdom, the body and mind will tend to purge themselves of these toxins. The detoxification process can appear as colds and flu, upper respiratory symptoms, skin or intestinal or other severe symptoms.

Sometimes bad dreams or bouts of the "blues" are signs of the mind detoxifying. Sometimes we need to slow down and let ourselves purge. When the symptoms persist, it is a sign we have high amounts of toxicity in our system. For example, ongoing depression, catarrh or dermatitis are our body's/mind's messages that we need to correct the errors of living that filled us with toxins.

If we are wise, pay attention to the minor issues that come up and change our behavior accordingly, we need never become seriously ill.

#2 If You Do Get Sick, Don't Go See Anyone

We go to see another person to heal us because of our tendency to look outside of ourselves to find an answer for a problem within. When we go to someone else, that interaction often gets in the way of doing what our body is desperately trying to do — get us to pay attention.

We believe that if we find the right doctor, all we need to do is turn over responsibility for our health, follow orders, and we will be basically healthy. This process is giving our power over to someone else. It is saying that we do not posses the wisdom to do for ourselves what it takes to be healthy. It is saying that we are not responsible for ourselves.

We proclaim we have to go to some expert who knows than we about the bodies we live in 24/7. It is saying that we do not trust ourselves to make decisions about what to do to stay well. It engages a false belief that we must inevitably become sick and broken down, but if we have the right experts around, they can fix us like our mechanic can fix our car. It ignores a fundamental truth that only we can perform routine maintenance on our bodies. Only we can care for ourselves and maintain our health. Our doctor/healer/acupuncturist/chiropractor/homeopath/whatever cannot sleep, drink water, exercise for us. Only we can keep ourselves healthy.

Health practitioners, myself included, are in the business of selling products and services. Revenue is generated best, like in all businesses, through repeat customers. It is in the best business interest of practitioners to never actually heal patients, just to make them feel better while we are seeing them, and to feel noticeably less well when we stop. Patients then triumphantly tell all of their friends how good they feel now that they are going to see Dr. X and that their friends should go too. Chiropractors are (sometimes unjustifiably) notorious for this.

The truth is that spinal and other joint and visceral manipulation is a powerful and effective healing technique, but if we don't do our work at home, it cannot fix us. We must do our exercise, stretches, change our diet, etc., in order to heal.

The medical/industrial establishment uses hype, the power of conventional institutions and a huge advertising budget to get us to keep coming back. M.D.s tell us that horrible things are going to happen if we do not take the prescribed pills for the rest of our lives. They convince us that there is a fundamental flaw in our previously perfect body system, and because we don't actually heal, we now have to keep coming back for follow-up appointments. They sell us virtual blindfolds and earplugs (in the form of medication) that let us stop seeing and hearing what our body and instinctual wisdom is, in increasingly loud ways, trying to tell us — straighten up and fly right. Unlike chiropractors, acupuncturists and naturopaths who, as a part of routine practice are *trained* to teach us how to take better care of ourselves, it is a rare M.D. who knows more than to tell us to quit smoking and get some exercise and maybe work on how we eat. Even rarer is an M.D. who has the predilection to do so.

Are acupuncturists and herbalists and naturopaths and other time-honored practitioners any better? The very fact that we go to someone else at all is saying to ourselves that we are lost and lack the power to heal our own bodies. If that is our true state, then we must go get help. In most cases, whatever ails us is reversible by following the messages we receive from God through our bodies' desires, emotions and intuition. We need to believe and act on the understanding that the healthiest way to live — as God/Nature designed us — is the easiest way to live.

Let's release the illusion that taking care of ourselves is somehow difficult or next to impossible. Why would God/Nature design a life form in such a way that it is more difficult to properly take care of it than not? If so, my bet is that that species is up next in the line for extinction. I know this can be a radical idea because so often to take care of ourselves in a natural way means that we must change our relationship to society and family. Do we really believe that making changes that are better for our individual health, can be bad for the planet as a whole?

My advice is that if you go to see someone else, only go with the commitment to change the behavior that got you there in the first place. Only go in to see someone if you already have an idea what the cause is, and you have started changing your behavior. Do your research first. Then only go to a professional who understands the behavioral cause of your problem, and who can help you change that behavior permanently.

#3 If You Go See Someone, Don't Go See An M.D.

Allopathic (standard Western) medicine — despite its huge, complex body of knowledge and its often-incomprehensible terminology and technology (even to those who practice it) — is actually quite simple.

Basically, it is like this: With some exceptions, the symptom is the problem. Using modern chemistry, metabolic processes are blocked (poisoned), and thus the symptom and the problem have been treated. The symptom, or the blood pressure, or the lab result or the x-ray result, etc., is the problem. Stop the symptom or reverse the lab finding, and the problem is gone? Not. Little or no consideration is given to the person's lifestyle and relationship to the world and to spirit as the origin of the problem. No consideration is given to the family situation or that of the greater society that is exploitive, and that prevents us from taking care for ourselves. Even less attention is given to preventing the problem from recurring. No surprise, it is common belief among M.D.s that patients cannot and will not change their behavior to heal themselves or to stay well.

But why do we have symptoms in the first place? Symptoms are God's way of letting us know we are out of alignment with our natural way of doing things. Symptoms are there to get us to pay attention. Pain is just another symptom that follows more subtle symptoms preceding it in the progression of the dis-ease. Stopping the symptom by itself, in the vast majority of the time, is counter productive for our healing. Our symptoms are our guides to re-establishing normal healthy behavior patterns.

In general, unless you have reached a severe crisis state and are looking out upon the abyss of death or disability, it is best to avoid the paradigm of allopathic medicine. Other "holistic" healing practices attempt to elucidate underlying patterns of disharmony, and by adjusting the spirit and body's function (with prayer or ritual, medication, hands on, movement, needles, heat, etc.), restore balance. If the holistic practitioner is practicing well, he or she will prescribe changes in lifestyle and relationship to the environment and work world. Holistic practitioners, unlike all but a miniscule portion of allopathic physicians, if doing their job, intend to motivate you to change your life.

Sometimes to actually do what your intuition and body tell you to do to heal is in fact a radical act that threatens the class and political nature of society. How many of us know we are in jobs, neighborhoods, relationships that make us sick? We drink water, breathe air and eat tainted food that makes us sick.

Our social condition as a consequence of our mental enslavement needs little elaboration here except to say that to date, functional political white supremacy is alive and well. This manifests in relatively poor health for Afrikans in the U.S. by all measured indices.[20] Political action may be the most rational response to many conditions causing our dis-eases. It is exceedingly rare to find the institution of orthodox medicine leading an initiative for social, political or economic change in conditions that clearly cause our dis-ease.

Standard medicine, as a major institution of society, is in place to reproduce, re-create and legitimize the existing order of society. No major institution in society actively antagonizes any other. Medicine is no different from the judiciary, legislative, military, banking, clergy, police, prison, entertainment or educational institutions. These institutions are in place to maintain the status quo.

When we realize we are natural vegetarians and stop eating animals, what will happen to the beef, poultry, dairy, fast-food, pharmaceutical, medical supply and hospital industries? That's right — they go out of business. What will happen when we refuse to work ourselves to death in dangerous and toxic jobs, and refuse to buy and consume stuff we really don't need? What happens when we refuse to have our neighborhoods serve as toxic waste dumps that affluent whites would not tolerate? There are major vested interests in our unhealthy lifestyle and they protect their interests well!

The institution of standard allopathic medicine, despite what many of us view as irrational in its approach to getting us well, when viewed from a political and economic perspective is actually quite rational as an institution of society. It tends and is intended to maintain the status quo. How often do we hear our physician tell us we need to quit our job that is stressing us out and making us sick and go into business for ourselves? Not too often, as we would lose our medical insurance and be unable to keep seeing the physician. To do so en masse would mean a loss in profit for the health care industry and a fundamental change in the exploitive nature of the relationship of business and industry to its workers.

It should come as no surprise despite over $100 billion spent for research on AIDS that we have no cure but only increasingly expensive treatment. As the gatekeepers and the demand drivers of the medical/industrial complex, doctors often act unwittingly as the front men, for a self-serving industry that seeks to maintain a constant low-level state of dis-ease. Just as the military seeks to maintain a constant state of war, there is no financial benefit to the medical pharmaceutical industry complex to actually cure AIDS (or any other chronic disease for that matter). There is too much profit to be gained by treating it. The same is true for hypertension, diabetes, arthritis, cancer — and the list goes on. Don't expect a business that reaps profits from you having a problem, to come up with a solution for you no longer having that problem. It is not in their best interest. What is in their best interest is to convince you that you need them to keep that problem "under control." Best if they can convince you that in order to keep that problem under control or to manage it, you must keep seeing them and keep using their products, or the products only they have the ability to authorize you to use "for the rest of your life."

Why are we so naive as to believe that although they state they have an oath ("Hippocratic vs. hypo-critic"), medicine as a profession and industry somehow operates on a different set of ethics than do all other industries?

#4 If You Go See An M.D., Don't Go See A Surgeon

There is an old adage: When one has a hammer in one's hand everything looks like a nail. Surgeons make their living doing surgery. The billing structure of medicine means that surgeons get paid large sums of money for the surgical procedure itself and very little for preliminary visits or follow up. Helping a person change their behavior so they will ultimately not need surgery is neither in a surgeon's financial best interest, nor is it within their range of training or experience. Referring the patient to an alternative practitioner who could possibly treat the condition without surgery is not what most surgeons will do. Their tendency is to cut first, think later.

Are we willing to accept never being entirely normal again after surgery? Cutting into the body permanently alters anatomy from its normal state. Removing parts of the internal organs renders the body unable to properly function or at least to optimally function, since all parts of the body are there for a reason. (Many of us have been told that the tonsils and appendix are vestigial organs and not needed. I don't buy that! God gave us just what we need, to do what we need to do.) Surgeons know this is true. Anyone who suggests otherwise to us is prevaricating.

I have on multiple occasions heard surgeons tell patients after having their gallbladder removed, that they can eat normally. A functioning gallbladder is necessary to properly digest a fatty meal. Once the gallbladder is removed, we must change the way we eat, especially since it is likely that we already eat a fatty diet that is the cause of most gallbladder disease.

Occasionally we ignore our body's messages, and fail to change our behavior and properly care for ourselves, continuing in our unhealthy patterns for long periods of time, to the point where death in hours is imminent without surgical intervention. Well at that point, gentlemen, sharpen your scalpels.

But until then, rare is the case where non-surgical intervention is not preferred and usually it is more effective. For example: there is overwhelming data[21] that show diet and lifestyle changes are more effective than surgery in treating coronary artery disease by every criterion of measurement. With non-surgical intervention, you don't end up with wires holding your chest together, and scars up and down your legs, with a high risk of having suffered brain damage from being on the heart-lung machine while your heart was stopped during surgery. Traditional Chinese medicine is more effective for the treatment of almost all gynecological dis-eases than Western surgical care. Only rarely is spinal surgery both truly indicated and as effective as movement and manual therapy.

Sure, I expect criticisms and that is OK. We can debate. But the fact remains — why would we do something that permanently alters the anatomy before we have really tried every other possible option, and resumed/started caring for our bodies fully in the natural way? We must take responsibility for caring for ourselves and get busy with it. Surgery does not, and seeks not to, address the cause of a problem. Witness the high rate of repeat coronary bypass surgeries. The underlying pattern of disharmony is not addressed and the problem usually recurs in an altered, identical or more severe form.

#5 If You Go See A Surgeon, Don't Go See One At A Teaching Hospital

In surgical training programs, witness the burned-out and jaded interns and residents referring to patients as their "surgical problem." Overhear a typical directive from senior resident to his intern — "I just admitted an appy*, finish your scut** and get down to the OR. I need you to scrub on this case." People are reduced from spiritual beings to diseased internal organs.

*In this usage "appy" means a person suffering from acute appendicitis.
**Scut is the day to day repetitive and tedious or odious work in the hospital that.

Surgical training requires residents to get practice in each type of operation. In fact, they have logbooks of operations that they must keep and submit for certification. This training is especially brutal and demanding. To be eligible for board certification, a surgeon in training must have performed a quota of each type of procedure in that specialty. Doctors will sometimes perform an operation that could be delayed or treated non-surgically — in order to meet that quota. Getting the numbers in is a reality. So the norm among surgical residents is severe sleep deprivation. Would you like someone cutting on you who is learning and has had neither lots of practice, nor a good night's sleep?

Surgical residency programs are very competitive. Only about 12 to 25 percent of interns starting surgical residency programs will finish. Residency programs are designed so that a good chunk of residents must be cut each year. Often the doctor who survives the cut is the most competitive and obsequious and not necessarily the most compassionate. Don't believe me? Go to a university hospital and ask.

Let us not forget the sordid history of surgical "science." This often criminally unconscionable past aggression on the bodies of Afrikans was well documented in the book "Medical Apartheid" by Harriet Washington. Forced, unauthorized sterilizations, hysterectomies for "hysteria," and brain surgery for mental illness, are among the dozens of procedures done often on poor and illiterate Black "patients."

There are many still commonly performed surgical procedures that are lacking scientific evidence as to their effectiveness, which were developed on Black people without true informed consent. No doubt some if not most of the procedures performed today will later be viewed as draconian when it becomes common knowledge that — given today's safe and effective treatment alternatives — they are not only unnecessary but harmful. All this stuff occurred in teaching hospitals under the guise of "science." Yes, they do continue to experiment on us in the operating room. Would you like these same sleepy doctors assisting a professor of surgery in performing new and experimental operations on you, the outcome of which is uncertain?

Despite this, I am not anti-surgery. In its proper role, surgical care is truly miraculous. But the last place I want to be is on an operating room table. If I am there, I know it is the only place I can be if I want to survive, or later function somewhat normally.

Remember and follow Adage # 1 Don't Get Sick. Do that by following the rule book and user guide installed at birth. Pay attention now to what our bodies are telling us. Know that our bodies are whole perfect and complete. Cooperate with our perfection by taking care of ourselves every day in every way.

Affirmation: I have everything I need to heal anything in me right now. I have the wisdom to know and to understand everything I need to be healthy all of my life. I care for my body, mind and soul and it responds with vibrant, enduring health.

The Rule Book And User Guide For Healthy Living

If you don't have time to heal, you get the time to die. — Akan/Twi

As a species, we Homo sapiens have been around for about a million years. That is 30,000 to 50,000 generations. We know that "civilization" has been around for maybe 100,000 years, or about 3,000-5,000 generations. We know our collective, ancestral memory goes back at least that far. When we incarnated into this life, we accepted this consciousness as ours. It operates on a daily basis as intuition and inner vision. Our intuition, which appears as immediate comprehension or cognition, is one of the main ways God talks to us. Like the insight of other animals, our "inner vision" guides us on our path.

Ancestral Memory

On a subconscious level, our ancestral wisdom is in continuous effect. We embody our ancestral memories of what we must do to stay alive and to stay healthy. We instinctively know what plants to eat and when. We instinctively know how to pay attention to our appetite and wisely choose foods that bring forth life energy. But because our culture has strayed so far from the truth of who we are, this knowledge is unavailable to us, for the most part, on a conscious level. We have unlearned the truth and have replaced it with "scientific" information that changes with the whims of commerce and technology. Our bodies, however, have been essentially biologically consistent for tens of thousands of generations. Traditionally,

Afrikan people have used divination and other spiritual means to tap into our ancestral wisdom. Part of our healing from the Maafa will be to reconnect with this ancestral wisdom. This is called re-Afrikanization.

We Have Perfect Health

Perfect health is coded into our ancestral consciousness. It is very much a state of mind and a system of beliefs. Life comes with what I call a rule book and user guide built in. In all animals, including humans, this rule book and user guide is called instinct. Also encoded is memory of the consequences of not following our rule book and user guide. We cannot escape these consequences, nor do I believe on a spiritual level we should want to. As human beings with advanced intellect, we think we can fake it by using our medicine, surgery, supplements, vitamins and healing techniques — ancient or contemporary. But we know, and deep down we know that we know, that if we do not cooperate with our ancestral living wisdom, we will have predictable consequences. We subconsciously know what these consequences are. We cannot transcend these consequences, unless we are fully aware of and in alignment with the full body of ancestral wisdom.

We each seek enlightenment, but it is unattainable by those who habitually break the rules. For example, we subconsciously know the consequences of not exercising or sleeping. Some of our distant ancestors tried to get away with not moving their bodies or sleeping regularly. We try to pretend we don't have to sleep regularly, drink adequate water, breathe properly, wash our bodies, etc. We know deep down inside that no matter how we try to fool ourselves — or try to "fix" ourselves with modern technology or ancient healing arts — we still know that if we don't take care of ourselves properly, we will endure specific consequences.

Cooperating With Our Abundance

We must cooperate with our abundance. Can we expect a bountiful garden if we do not water and till the soil? We know that if we pray for a new home, we must be prepared to move into it. We know that if we pray for a perfect partner and lover, we must be prepared when they show up. We know if we pray for a new car, we must learn how to drive. Can we expect our cars to run properly if we do not keep them fueled, lubricated and tuned?

Remember: The rules have not changed in hundreds of thousands of years. They are the same now as they were for our distant ancestors. If we are in dis-ease and are healing, this is even more consequential. We intuitively know we have not been following our ancestrally encoded rule book and user guide, and we are now experiencing the consequences. In our modern technological society, we spend the early part of our lives forgetting this knowledge of life that God instilled in our collective consciousness.

Let's go about remembering today. The following are the basics. I have ordered the rules, the first ones being the most urgent, but not necessarily the most important.

Nana Kwaku's Life Rules For Human Beings

We Must Breathe Properly.

We Must Drink Water.

We Must Rest, Sleep And Dream.

We Must Eat Wisely, Individualized To Our Body Constitution.

We Must Perform Certain Acts We Call Hygiene.

We Must Not Poison Ourselves.

We Must Move Our Bodies Wisely, Individualized To Our Body Constitution.

We Must Expose Ourselves To The Sun.

We Must Engage In Complementary Relations With Others.

We Must, Through Knowledge Of Self, Respect, Align, And Harmonize Ourselves With The Natural World. We Must Live In The Practice Of Maat.

We Must Connect With Our God Essence And To Our Ancestral Wisdom Through Spiritual Work And Practice.

We Must Be On Our Purpose And Use Our Divinely Gifted Genius In Service To The World.

We Must Participate In The Growing/Raising Of The Children.

We Must Actively Reclaim Our Afrikanity And Culture.

We Must Have A Habitual Practice Of Loving Kindness.

We Must Engage In Right Livelihood.

There are consequences for failing to follow the rules as set forth in your rule book, the understanding and particulars of which are held in our collective consciousness. God lovingly enforces the rules for us by giving us sensations, feelings, thoughts and premonitions. These are what I call lessons.

Lessons are given initially very subtly and gently. Lessons are given in increasingly firm and purposeful ways until learned. Eventually, if the behavior is not modified, the lessons become painful and prevent us from functioning well. God and our ancestors are always on duty, lessons are repeated and amplified until learned — and the rules followed at all times. Most of us believe that the enforcement/penalties/consequences for disregard of these rules is a normal part life, such as age-related degeneration, adult onset diabetes, hypertension, arthritis, vision and hearing loss, impotence, and the like. No! We don't have to get traffic tickets, we don't have to go to jail, our cars never have to break down and we don't have to get sick, rundown or debilitated.

These and other dis-ease states are lessons not learned when given in more subtle forms. We subconsciously know what these lessons are teaching us through our ancestral wisdom. Our ancestors have experienced them before. We cannot get around this. Although our intellect oftentimes tries hard to ignore this truth, we know on a deep intuitive level what will come of failing to follow the rules. Some of us have forgotten who and what we are, and what we agreed to when we accepted this incarnation. We think the rules do not apply to us. We are surprised, hurt, mad at God, feel betrayed, etc., when the rules are enforced. We plead and we bargain with God, when God is only reminding us about what we agreed to do in the first place — love and care for our bodies, the vessels of our soul.

Many of us pay large sums of money to talented and often effective health practitioners. We think they can heal us because they have gone to school and possess greater knowledge, wisdom and talent. We think they can sell us something or do something to us that lets us ignore God's messages to us through sensations and intuition. Often we feel better transiently, only to have our symptoms reappear when we stop going or taking medication. We must cooperate with our healing. Why do we spend so much money and still have ill health? We must follow the rules. Let's not waste our time and money on good healing arts to stay sick! Let's pay attention to the messages we continually get from God through our bodies, hearts, and minds. Let's cooperate with our abundant health. Let's heal now and stay well!

1. We Must Breathe Properly

Breathing is so important that it is the one thing we will do without giving it any thought. Without breathing we will die or suffer permanent brain injury within 10 minutes. Breathing is automatic. Or is it? If we intentionally try to not breathe, we will soon pass out and start breathing automatically again. My experience has shown me that few of us breathe properly.

Because breathing is so closely associated with speech and emotions, emotional blocks also cause breathing blocks. How often when you are stressed do you find yourself holding your breath, only to release it with a big sigh when the stress is released? As you hold your breath, toxins build up in the blood. Carbon dioxide is not exhaled and oxygen is not taken in. The blood acidifies and puts strain on the kidneys to maintain the acid-base balance in the blood.

Our sedentary lifestyle discourages many of us from taking deep cleansing breaths. In Sanskrit, "prana" means breath. Pranayama yoga is a large part of kundalini and tantra yoga, and its practice revolves around controlling the breath and using it to cultivate and enhance energy. Pranayama helps us exercise and tone our most important physical activity — to breathe.

Here is what mindful and intentional breathing can do — when you are anxious or tense, try taking ten fast, complete, deep breaths in a row. Breathe in through the nose and out through the mouth. See how this conscious breathing will cleanse the emotions and relax you.

Let us never do anything that will harm the body's ability to breathe. Smoking cigarettes is the most harmful thing you can do to your health and is one of the most life-denying activities normally thought to be pleasurable. I am dedicated and focused on helping my patients actually heal. I am less focused on treating the illness than with identifying and empowering my patients to remove the cause of their illnesses. This is why if I have a patient who smokes and asks for help with any other problem, I will address the smoking problem first. Smoking is so damaging to every process in the body. Many of the chemicals inhaled are deadly cell poisons that inhibit or block the body's mechanisms from healing from all other illnesses. If you smoke — quit now. Get help.

2. We Must Drink Water

Water is essential to almost every biochemical activity of life. In general, a person can survive from one to ten days without water, depending on the temperature, humidity and availability of shade and exertion level. If you go one day without water or other fluids (including in food), I guarantee you will feel miserable or worse. In modern American city life, water is taken for granted.

How do you know you are getting enough water? I generally recommend drinking enough to keep you producing urine frequently and that the color is very pale, almost clear white. That will ensure no matter how much activity you are doing or what the temperature is, your body is getting enough fluid to perform bodily functions and eliminate toxins.

Clean water is essential too. Due to agricultural and industrial pollution, most tap water contains significant amounts of toxins. A good water filter is one of the best investments you can make for your health.

3. We Must Rest, Sleep And Dream

Do not fall asleep in your enemy's Dream. — John Edgar Wideman

On average, a human can go 200 hours before dying from sleep deprivation. During sleep, the body, mind and spirit regenerates, and most healing occurs.

Dreaming is also important. During dreamtime we are often given messages from the Divine. It is the time when we process toxic unconscious thoughts, feelings and images that have been absorbed during the day or earlier in life. It is the time when premonitions are received that are later interpreted as deja vu.

Sleep deprivation is probably the most common cause of injuries and accidents in this country. It is also one of the most common causes of academic failure in children and adults. It is one of the most common reasons for failure to heal and one of the reasons that the hospital is one of the worst places to recover from illness or injury — few people get good rest while in the hospital.

How can you tell whether you get enough sleep? You will have had dreams during the night. You can wake up in the morning spontaneously and have no need for alarms or stimulants. You go through the day alert and attentive.

4. We Must Eat Wisely, Individualized To Our Body Constitution

There is no medicine as active as good food. — Igbo

Without doubt, what you put into your mouth has profound effects on your health. You quite literally are what you eat. If you eat junk, you become junk. Huge amounts of disease come directly from eating improperly. Sadly, the vast majority of the world's population does not eat in alignment with natural law.

As is described elsewhere in this book, it has been exhaustively and conclusively shown that the consumption of animal products leads directly to the majority of health problems from which we suffer. A growing body of evidence supports the argument that eating cooked food is not the best for human health and is sometimes outright damaging. Changing the way we eat has an immediate, discernible effect on how we feel.

These effects are most easy to identify and can be documented in a food journal. See the Appendix on how to create a food journal.

For most people, the key to optimal health is tailoring their food consumption to their body's constitution. The fat/carbohydrate/protein ratio for optimum functioning varies, even between siblings. Most people are aware that certain foods don't "sit well" with them.

There are both ancient and modern tools for discerning a person's body constitution. Most of this information is available in books or by consulting a dietitian versed in the relation between diet and body constitution. However, the best way is by self-experimentation and careful observation of the effect of each food you consume. It is the surest way to find which foods work for you.

5. We Must Perform Certain Acts We Call Hygiene

The abscess heals when opened. — Thonga

Cleanliness is next to godliness. We associate dirt and filth with poor health for good reason. As crucial as keeping the body clean, keeping your environment around you clean has a profound effect on one's health. Most communicable diseases are preventable by proper hygiene and sanitation. Introducing public sanitation measures into a community is by far the single most important factor (other than social change) in reducing or eliminating a disease. Clean water, proper waste disposal and sanitation are more important than medication and vaccinations in promoting the public health.

In developed areas, the problem is not inadequate hygiene but improper hygiene. Today we have lost sight of how important it is to naturally clean ourselves amidst the storm cloud of merchandising of artificial products. Few of the products available in the corner drugstore or supermarket have been adequately tested on human beings, especially for long-term effects. Some products routinely used — especially by Black women on their hair — have well-known adverse effects on health; scalp burns from hot combs and lye, rashes and acne from skin cosmetics, and cancer caused by the hair dyes and bleaches.

It is amazing to me how few of these products actually do anything positive. Other than using soap where hair grows on the body, if you are eating right, nothing other than clean water is needed to beautify the skin and hair.

Even more critical than proper physical hygiene and sanitation is mental and spiritual hygiene. The thoughts we think and the information we expose ourselves to have a profound effect on our health. Negativity begets negativity. If we are around toxic people, their negative attitudes and energy vibrations rub off on us. If we watch endless television crime dramas, we will become infected by violent, life-denying energy. This is especially important for mothers and pregnant women. Children, even those unborn, are most susceptible to these influences.

The mass media tends to inculcate European values and culture. It has the infectious yurugu virus.[22] The more we take in, the more whitenized[23] and falsified[24] our consciousness becomes. Many of us think we are immune to these effects. The owners of the media-industrial complex study diligently how to affect viewers' thinking and subconscious mind. It is best to avoid the mass media, except where active simultaneous deconstruction of what is on the screen is being done by conscious elders — mature individuals who did not grow up on the constant diet of mass media mind control. Elders who have de-whitenized and verified their Afrikan self-consciousness. We all are affected by the mass media in one way or another — and the Internet is no better.

Just by controlling the topics and the range of discussion, the barons of the media influence what we think about. They are expert in forming attitudes and feelings that control our behavior. Most notable is the overwhelming advertising pressure from the meat and dairy industries. Then along come drug companies, advertising products that are supposed to counter the effects of the wanton disregard for our dietary health promoted in the media. The desacralized, anti-Afrikan and hyper-sexualized pansexual "anything is fair game" slant of the media make it difficult if not impossible for us to engage in positive behaviors. By sheer repetition, we have come to accept the assumptions on which the media bases its lies (9/11 = al-Qaida, HIV = AIDS.) Our natural Afrikan mind and way of thinking has been replaced with that of our conquerors. Our conceptual basis of reality becomes distorted and diseased. Our consciousness becomes that of our enemies, and we no longer act in our own best interest. This is evident when we see our children emulating the often-vulgar, materialistic and misogynistic behavior on BET and other media.

6. We Must Not Poison Ourselves

Many of us are committing slow suicide by the poisons we ingest. Tobacco, caffeine, alcohol, drugs of all types, environmental toxins such as bug spray, certain cleaning products, foods contaminated with pesticides and herbicides, are all known to be harmful to our bodies and minds. The spiritual subtext we are saying to ourselves and to God is that we place more value in the pleasure or ease these things give us than in the sanctity of our sacred body temple. We symbolically defecate in the corner of the temple, the temple God gave us to house our spirit at birth.

This temple was designed to last and house our spirit for our lifetime and allow us to do the work we were born to do. Those of us who attend church could not begin to imagine doing to the church building what we do to our bodies. Perhaps we should begin to fear what God will do to us for soiling our own body temple as much as we would fear soiling the church.

Eat organic vegetarian food to avoid bio-magnification. Bio-magnification occurs when an animal eats contaminated foods and the toxins build up in bodily tissues. When another animal eats the contaminated animal, it receives bio-magnified toxins. This is why many carnivorous species are endangered — they eat DDT, other pesticides and heavy metals that their prey ingested. This also explains why one study found the breast milk of meat-eating women had 35 times the pesticides as that of vegetarian women.[25]

7. We Must Move Our Bodies Wisely, Individualized To Our Body Constitution

Just about everybody knows that you cannot be serious about your health if you do not exercise. But what kind of exercise and how much? If your goal is health and not qualifying for gladiator-type activities, then you exercise to feel good and to keep feeling good. Looking good will come as a byproduct of feeling good.

People often come to me to lose weight. I ask them why they are trying to lose weight. My belief is that if you have the right pattern of diet and exercise, you will naturally migrate to the proper weight for your body constitution.

There are two types of exercise, internal and external. What most Westerners call exercise is external exercise, which is meant to allow you to move and expend energy.

Internal exercise is designed to cultivate the inner workings of the body. It is designed to cultivate and build qi, enhance respiration, digestion and elimination. It is designed to ensure the free and easy flow of energy through the body and to calm and center the mind.

Both external and internal exercise are important. If your internal function is good, then your ability to expend energy is good. If your internal body function is constrained or weakened, the ability to perform physical activities is diminished. Tai chi, qi gong and yoga are the best-known forms of internal exercise. Internal exercise should be taught in childhood and the practice continued daily throughout life, regardless of external exercise. The benefits of internal exercise are many and the risks are few.

Because we must get around in the world and on occasion must physically defend ourselves, external exercise is also essential.

I place the goals of external exercise and its benefits as a) balance; b) flexibility and pliability of the joints and muscles; c) core strength and posture; d) endurance; e) overall strength.

Balance. Because we stand and walk erect, the first thing we must do is keep from falling over. Many young people take this for granted. The elderly often list fear of falling down as one of the primary reasons they avoid outdoor activities. This is with good reason. Hip and other fractures often lead to suffering and death in the elderly. Falling is a dangerous proposition for all ages. Falling and hitting your head on a hard surface is enough to kill you. This is why it is of crucial importance for all bicycle riders to wear a helmet, no matter how fast or slow they ride. Having good balance is key.

Flexibility. Because we do fall, it is important that our muscles and joints be flexible and pliable to absorb shock. Flexibility (and avoiding of reckless behavior and dangerous sports) is the key to remaining injury-free. It is also the key to remaining pain-free as you age.

Core Strength and Posture. Because we stand erect, core strength and posture are necessary to hold the body upright. Keeping the vertebra properly stacked upon each other is essential for the proper action of respiration and digestion. Integrity of the spinal musculature and abdominal musculature and its proper coordination and tone ensures this. Many doctors teach sit-ups as the key exercise. Properly done, sit-ups are a great way to strengthen and tone the abdominal wall muscles rectus abdominus*, but they do not effectively tone the obliques* and transversus abdominus*. Often ignored is the quadratus lumborum* as a posture-maintaining muscle*. Hatha yoga and Pilates are excellent for building core strength. This is why we offer instruction in both at our center in Atlanta.

* All of these muscles are part of the abdominal wall.

Endurance. Those of us preoccupied with our appearance often overlook endurance. However, being fit has to do with not just looking good but being able to maintain physical output long enough to get done what you are doing or getting to where you need to go or to get away from danger. The most important defensive skill is running. No one can defeat you in a fight if they cannot catch you. There is always going to be someone stronger than you. They may have a gun or a knife. But they cannot defeat you if you run away. Raw speed is important for the first 100 yards or so. But after that it is endurance that counts. More battles are won because of the army's ability to sustain their output than by how many pounds the soldiers can bench press.

Overall Strength. Speed does not mean that strength is unimportant. Having the ability to push away or pull up or lift your weight or that of your family member is a very important survival ability. Muscle strength also supports the joints and protects them from injury. Having good muscle mass and strength is important for doing everything else. However, if one focuses on balance, posture, flexibility and endurance, one will develop strength in the process. Weight training done intelligently is an excellent activity, however most people need only to do calisthenics and simple gymnastic movements such as pulls-ups, push-ups and squats, etc. More than that is only helpful if you are competing in an activity that requires speed and power. Soldiers need to be strong but not at the expense of the other aspects of fitness.

8. We Must Expose Ourselves To The Sun

All life can trace its origin to the sun. It is solar energy that warms the planet. It provides the energy that plants use to grow. This process is known as photosynthesis. What is not commonly known is that human beings also are able to store solar radiation energy as melanin pigment. When melanin is formed in the skin during the process of tanning, energy is stored in the melanin molecule. Photo-radiation energy absorbed through the skin is used to build melanin molecules. Energy is released when the melanin is later broken down and used for other purposes. Vitamin D is produced in the skin when the skin is exposed to sunlight. Vitamin D is clearly essential for life. Outdoors, we are exposed to solar and cosmic radiation. Without sunlight we become depressed and weak.

9. We Must Engage In Complementary Relations With Others

We need other people in our life to be fulfilled. The worst punishment other than torture or execution is solitary confinement. A basic and fundamental principle is that we have a complementary exchange with those around us. We must interact in a reciprocal way that is mutually beneficial.

The choice of spouse and who to have children with are some of the most important decisions a person will make. Many of us have incorrectly made this choice based on emotion alone more than once. In the Western-influenced world, it is sad that this decision is taken so lightly and is made with so little foresight and wisdom. We must learn to judge potential partners by the content of their character and the compatibility of temperament and life purpose, not by the chemical reaction of hormones and physical attraction, and not by the superficial value system of the European.

Traditionally, prior to the colonial imposition of foreign courtship practices, families married one another when two adults came together as a couple. The family elders, having wisdom, could discern and understand the young adults' strengths, weakness, proclivities and purposes in life. With wisdom unclouded by physical attraction and hormones, they could best judge whether the two young adults complemented one another.

The success of a man or a woman (and their children) is directly related to the success of their marriage. When you procreate, the two lineages are forever bound and you create a lifelong relationship. If you are wise, you will be very careful about who you have sex with. Consider very carefully avoiding conception, even after marriage, until it is clear you and your spouse are fully compatible and share life purpose and parenting philosophies.

As a result of the Maafa and our enslavement, we were sometimes conditioned to breed like chattel animals without regard to the offspring that result. We could expect that those offspring would often be taken from us and sold. Some of us have continued to behave sexually like slaves. Especially some of our most mentally enslaved males who attempt to impregnate as many females as possible, without regard to the children who result.

Relations must be reciprocal, a natural balance of giving and receiving. In Afrikan culture, there is a reciprocal order to personal and community relations. We naturally give back to those who give to us — not as a mechanism for keeping a balance sheet, but because it is the right thing to do. The idea that one can exploit another for energy and time is not our way, although it has become increasingly prevalent in our communities.

Relations should be complementary. The strengths of one person balances the weakness of the other and vice versa. We should seek partners who have skills and talents we do not have to complete the skill set within a couple.

A word about homosexuality. Prior to the Arab and European invasions, homosexuality was foreign to Afrikan people. In European culture, there is a long history of homosexual relations going back to the Greeks. The traditional Afrikan community was organized around the children. Fertility and child rearing were prized. Having children was an essential part of rising within the social structure and was expected of all priests and chiefs and, of course, queen mothers. Those who were unable or unwilling to participate in having children did not participate in all aspects of society. However, in Afrikan cultures there were rare individuals who posessed an abundance of energy of the opposite gender. There was an honored role in society for these people. They were not ostracized or excluded. However, sexual contact with a member of the same sex was not known.

A word about monogamy. The concept of monogamy is very different in traditional Afrikan culture than it is in European culture. Marital infidelity (dishonesty) was rare. If sex between two single people was practiced, it was a part of courtship and there was no secrecy or shame involved. Secondly, there was a distinct difference in how lineage was determined. Matrilinialism was the norm. The woman held equal if not more important power than that of the man. The wife was not the property of the husband. The decision to bring another wife into the family was traditionally that of the senior wife. If she and her husband felt that the family could benefit by having the skills and energy of another woman, or if there was a need to provide a husband to give children to a woman in the community that otherwise would not have the opportunity, the family could afford the cost, and there was a need to join the two families, she would instigate the marriage of another wife. Keep also in mind that in most Afrikan cultures there were many different forms of marriage, which may or may not involve sex or procreation. Sexual misconduct and rape were not a part of the Afrikan community in general, prior to the influx of Islam and Christianity. Thirdly there was no imperative[26] for recreational sexual conduct as there was in the West.

We have accepted a value system and behavioral norm of that of our conquering oppressors/enslavers. This has led us into much disorder within our families. Our traditional family structure led to successful, peaceful and harmonious organization of the community. It empowered and placed children and women at the center of the community. The rape, homosexuality and child molestation currently decimating our community were unknown. If we want to be healthy, we must have healthy families. There is only one logical conclusion to this dilemma — the modern Afrikan person must relearn and practice pre-colonial Afrikan ways of relating to each other.

There are several excellent guides to proper relations with the opposite sex. I recommend those by Yao Nyamekye Morris, "The Natural Blueprint For Relationships"; Ra Un Nefer Amen, "An Afrocentric Guide To A Spiritual Union"; Mwalimu Baruti, "Complementarity And The Sex Imperative" and "Homosexuality And The Efeminization Of The Afrikan Male."

10. We Must Respect, Align And Harmonize Ourselves With The Natural World. We Must Live In The Practice Of Maat[27]

Humans are the only animals that miss this concept. With the exception of many indigenous nations, in relation to the rest of the planet, we have become, as a species, like a cancer that expands, eats away and lays waste to the rest of the world. We grind away at the environment without regard to harmony or the future. Although this was a foreign concept to Afrika prior to our conquest, as a result of the Maafa, we too seem to believe that we can destroy at our whim anything or anyone we find around us. Harmonizing with the environment, fulfilling a niche in the ecosystem is something other animals and species do. Not us. Our species has no respect for our natural range in the environment. Instead, we have spread practically all over the globe. Our intellect has enabled us to override our common sense. It has gotten to the point where sense is not too common anymore.

The Forty-Two Negative Affirmations Of Maat

There are 42 divine principles of Maat. I have seen several slightly different versions. Here is one:

I Have Not Committed Sin.

I Have Not Committed Robbery With Violence.

I Have Not Stolen.

I Have Not Slain Men Or Women Without Cause.

I Have Not Stolen Food.

I Have Not Swindled Offerings.

I Have Not Stolen From God/Goddess.

I Have Not Told Lies.

I Have Not Carried Away Food.

I Have Not Cursed.

I Have Not Closed My Ears To Truth.

I Have Not Committed Sodomy.

I Have Not Made Anyone Cry.

I Have Not Felt Sorrow Without Reason.

I Have Not Assaulted Anyone.

I Have Not Been Deceitful.

I Have Not Stolen Anyone's Land.

I Have Not Been An Eavesdropper.

I Have Not Falsely Accused Anyone.

I Have Not Been Angry Without Reason.

I Have Not Seduced Anyone's Wife.

I Have Not Polluted Myself.

I Have Not Terrorized Anyone.

I Have Not Disobeyed The Law.

I Have Not Been Excessively Angry.

I Have Not Cursed God/Goddess.

I Have Not Behaved With Violence.

I Have Not Caused Disruption Of Peace.

I Have Not Acted Hastily Or Without Thought.

I Have Not Overstepped My Boundaries Of Concern.

I Have Not Exaggerated My Words When Speaking.

I Have Not Worked Evil.

I Have Not Used Evil Thoughts, Words Or Deeds.

I Have Not Polluted The Water.

I Have Not Spoken Angrily Or Arrogantly.

I Have Not Cursed Anyone In Thought, Word Or Deeds.

I Have Not Placed Myself On A Pedestal.

I Have Not Stolen What Belongs To God/Goddess.

I Have Not Stolen From Or Disrespected The Deceased.

I Have Not Taken Food From A Child.

I Have Not Acted With Insolence.

I Have Not Destroyed Property Belonging To God/Goddess.

11. We Must Connect With Our God Essence And To Our Ancestral Wisdom Through Spiritual Work And Practice

Ancestral wisdom unraveled, retraced, revised, and resurrected will promote the reclamation and re-ascension of our people. — Nsenga Warfield-Coppock

We are spiritual beings. We are born of the spirit and we return to spirit. The divine creative force that is present in our daily lives is known by many different names. And while there are many different religious faiths or expressions of this divine spiritual energy, they each are aimed at connecting to the Creator. Whether we call that creator God, Allah, Oludumare or Goddess, it is the same creative force. Each religious faith has found its own path to try to reach that force.

Our Afrikan ancestral spirituality is at the root of the world's religions. As we look back and study these roots, we can find the seeds of traditional Afrikan spirituality in other faith traditions. As Afrikan people today, we must recognize and remember that the religious traditions of our ancestors were stolen from us through colonization and the enslavement of our people. We did not give them up willingly or because they didn't work for us.

These ancestral traditions are still alive and well today. In Afrika, many people have shrines for their ancestors and family deities in their homes. They continue to participate in the ceremonies and practices as their families have for thousands of years. Some practice the traditional spirituality of Akan, Ifa or Voudon, etc., exclusively, while others do so alongside the newer Muslim or Christian religions. Here in the Americas, the traditions brought by the enslaved Afrikans were hidden under the façade of Catholicism forced upon them, to be expressed in Santeria, Candomble, Obeah, Haitian Voudo, and others found in the Caribbean and South and Central America. More Afrikans in the Americas are reaching back to reconnect to these traditions as practiced in the Diaspora and in the Motherland.

In addition, even those who are more traditionally Christian embody many of the roots of our Afrikan ways. "Getting the holy ghost," speaking in tongues, dancing, clapping, the call and response, pouring of libations, and many other worship characteristics often found in Black churches are reminiscent of our traditional Afrikan spiritual practices of ritual, celebration, possession and communion with the ancestors and deities.

Indigenous spiritual practices the world over place high regard on honoring and connecting with the ancestors. Recognizing our sacred duty to remain in balance with the Earth and those around us is also a vital aspect. Indigenous peoples involve the creator in all aspects of their lives. Divination is used to speak to and listen to the spirit world for guidance. These are our ways as Afrikans. We have been distracted by European ways.

Regardless of our religious path, it is important to remember that our ancestors live on in us, and live forward through our descendants. No matter which faith we follow, each of us has a personal connection to our ancestors and the divine. We can bring our ancestors' energy and wisdom into our daily lives by creating a special place to honor them in our homes. You may already have a place where you display photos of your ancestors. What you have created might be called an ancestor shrine or altar. By adding white candles, a white cloth, water in a crystal glass, and other objects that belonged to or remind us of our loved ones, you make this shrine more personal and more powerful. Each day you may prepare a small plate of food for your ancestors as an offering. Before you leave the house for the day, pour libations to your ancestors and the Creator. Offer a prayer of gratitude and reverence for the blessings in your life. Ask for their protection and assistance. These steps can help you to tap into a deep well of power, knowledge and guidance. The ancestors' wisdom speaks to us through our dreams and intuition. As we align our thoughts and our lives to this power, we may notice shifts occurring in our reality.

12. We Must Be On Our Purpose And Use Our Divinely Gifted Genius In Service To The World

In many ways I think this is the most important rule. Each of us is born with some kind of talent. We all have something that we do very well. Something that if nurtured becomes our natural genius. This is a gift from God and our ancestors on the occasion of our birth. We come to this planet for a purpose. We have divinely appointed work to do. We have our life's work. This is what we agreed to do prior to birth when we were enlisted by our ancestors and the Divine to do this work. We agreed to use this talent for good. We agreed to use this talent in service of our lineage, our community, our nation and the world. This is our purpose in life. When we are doing our true work, we are on purpose, we have the support and assistance of our ancestors and the Divine. Things seem to flow. The resources needed to do what we want seem to appear in our path. Time flows smoothly and quickly. We are productive. We need not make an effort or struggle to achieve our goals. Things occur with effortless ease. Work is fun and satisfying. We are at ease with those around us and are happy. This is being in the "zone".[28]

Sadly, most of us are not on purpose these days. Most of us have not found our true inborn genius. Most of us have been sold the idea that we are mediocre people and have little to contribute. We have been told that we might as well just put up with our lot in life, work hard and eke out an existence. We lack meaning in life. We go though our days with glimpses of happiness yet feel an emptiness and underlying sense of despair. We have no idea what this life is all about. This is what disease is all about. We are lacking ease. We lack our effortless ease. And we feel it.

Sometimes we fall into the abyss of despair and lose all ambition. We become depressed and angry with God for our miserable lot in life. We lose our drive to live and are on an increasingly slippery, meaningless slope to our grave. We engage in behaviors we know are negative and are damaging to our health. We are on a quest for death. We look for the answer in drugs, food-like substances, sex or thrill-seeking to temporarily quench that thirst for meaning — only to leave that "hole in our soul" even deeper than before. We desperately seek relief when the subconscious illusion of soul soothing inevitably wears off. We seek relief for this profound emptiness.

The Maafa is all about us being *off* purpose. As Afrikans, we have the oldest and greatest civilizations. We created and refined all the basic arts and practices that define culture, and these spread throughout the world. We were the original people in the original center of the world. For our enemies to conquer us, we had to lose sight of what we were doing. As a people we had to get off purpose. We had to lose sight of who and what and where and when we were. We somehow lost our direction and thus the backing of the Divine.

Those who would conquer us were and are acutely aware of this. This is why they first took our spiritual practice from us. They replaced it with religion that supported their ways, ethos and mythology. This is why they also took our language and customs, and to this day they mis-educate us into believing we did not have any meaningful or valuable customs. When they could not deny our ways, they vilified and demonized them. It was essential that we became and stayed alienated from ourselves. It was essential for our enslavers — and their heirs who benefit from our enslavement — that we never know who we really are. To continue to exploit us, it is essential that we stay off purpose and continue to be addicts — if not, we would bring to bear all the power of the universe to help us live our way.

God and our ancestors do not want us to live in an inferior, exploited state. Our ancestors and our deities use their power to help us stay strong and healthy as a people and a nation. We are each given a gift that they help us use to build healthy lives for our families, our communities, our nation and ourselves. This power cannot be defeated. It is the power of God helping us to do what we agreed to do when we were born.

This cycle operates on a level where we are unaware, even in the deepest throes of addiction. When we are on purpose, the hole in our soul fades away. Spirit offers clues to our purpose and reminders that we need to get back on our path all the time.

13. We Must Participate In The Raising Of The Children

We must be about the business of liberating the minds of Black children. In order for that to occur, the minds of all Blacks who interact with them must also be liberated. There is no other way. — Bobby E. Wright

To deculturalize Afrikan American children is, therefore, to deprive them of that which determines the way they think, feel and behave. — Felix Boateng

How many times have you heard "The children are our future"? Yet society doesn't function as if this were true. Supporting the healthy development of our Afrikan children is one of the most important jobs we have. All of the other rules in this book feed directly into this one. We need to take care of ourselves so that we are in optimal form to take on that task. We need to ensure that we are around well into our elder-hood to share the wisdom we have gained through our experiences. We need to model and share these life-giving rules with the younger generation so that they too will be strong and healthy.

So what does this have to do with your health? Afrikan culture recognizes that we cannot be healthy in isolation. We need a strong community where healthy lifestyle choices are seen as normal. This community reinforces and supports our health by providing the support, resources and environment we need. This community does not undermine and destroy us, as does the current mainstream white supremacist culture.

Ultimately a part of all Afrikans' purpose here in this life is to support our people and ensure that we continue on into the future. For most of us, this includes raising children of our own.

However, you don't have to be a parent or grandparent to help raise children and youth. I am sure you have also heard the saying, "It takes a village to raise a child." Children and youth need aunties and uncles, big brothers and sisters (both those related by marriage or blood and those tied by strong social bonds), teachers, coaches and other mentors, neighbors, community leaders — everyone has a responsibility to care for the children and to be mindful of the needs of children everywhere.

We cannot accomplish this vital job if we continue to let our children be raised and mis-educated by the media, mainstream schools and by a eurocentric, white supremacist society. We must take back the minds, bodies and souls of our people by taking back the minds of our children. We didn't get to our current state overnight. We wont get back to our divine place as a people overnight either. The children are the key. It may take seven or more generations to reach our destination. We must start now with this generation of children.

Fortunately there are a growing number of families and communities who have heard the call and are doing just this. They have unplugged their families from the matrix. They are homeschooling their children or sending them to Afrikan-centered schools that teach our history, literature, leadership, languages and culture. They are feeding their children healthy food and taking them to doctors who use natural healing rather than standard Western approaches. They have incorporated Afrikan spiritual and cultural practices into their daily lives. They involve their children in the community, expose them to wise elders and provide role models of strong, beautiful, proud Afrikan people. It is beautiful to be in the presence of these families, to see these children growing with a sense of pride and confidence that is often missing in other children. They are learning to love their Afrikanity, to recognize their worth, and to be able to see the matrix for what it is.

These families cannot operate in isolation. The schools need teachers and directors. They need spiritual leaders who perform rituals and ceremonies and a spiritual community for support. They need lawyers, accountants, physicians, real estate agents, and other professionals who are culturally Afrikan-oriented. They need artists and performers who create culturally relevant work, to share their talents and encourage young people to develop their own.

Afrikan children and families need us to be healthy. We need them to be healthy in order for us to be healthy. We are the village that it takes to raise our strong, proud, Afrikan-oriented children and youth. It takes us all.

14. We Must As Afrikan People Actively Reclaim Our Afrikanity And Culture

To go back to tradition is the first step forward. — Afrikan Proverb

There are few things in the world as dangerous as sleepwalkers. — Ralph Ellison

We must through the Sankofa process reclaim our Afrikanity and culture as Afrikan people. We are out of our right minds. We must realize that at the root of our trouble is the false belief that we do not have to be true to our deepest selves. Through the effects of over two thousand years of the imposition of foreign culture and mis-education, we have come to hold a false belief that our ancestors were either weak, stupid, primitive or betrayed us, or all of the above. It comes from a lie that we have been consistently indoctrinated into, from the earliest days of our enslavement and colonization — and it persists to this day. We still believe that we have little or nothing of value in our Afrikan culture that we need to regain or hold onto.

The doctrine of cultural Darwinism holds that because Europeans developed civilization last and because they have come to dominate the world, that their culture is the best and greatest product of evolution. Those that endorse (either implicitly or explicitly) cultural Darwinism believe Black/Afrikan/primitive people have an un-evolved nature, and we are stuck in our ancient ways. We falsely believe to advance, to have all that is fine and good in the world, Blacks must adopt modern (i.e., eurocentric) cultural norms. The fundamental lie of cultural Darwinism is even more strongly held than white supremacy. It is the most tightly held philosophy of Europeans. It is more fundamental to them than any other philosophy. It is essential to his continued domination of the world that people of color, especially Afrikans, must believe this also. It is European culture and ways (as well as their purported genetic superiority) that are supreme, causing them to naturally rise to the top. They have a manifest destiny[29] to rule the world. Consequently, cultural Darwinism mandates that for a person of color to attain some semblance of comfort and success, we must become as like the whites as we can.

We falsely believe we must whitenize.[30] We have been convinced that to be happy is to be like white. It is essential that we discard what is unique and powerful about us for white supremacy/domination to persist. It is essential that we behave, speak, dress, play, sleep, eat, talk, work, date, are born, die, heal, worship, teach, learn and settle conflict as do the white people. This ensures that the possible questions asked are constrained. And because the assumptions are within the context of European cultural norms, the solutions that logically ensue will ultimately benefit the Europeans at our expense.

That we are fundamentally different from them at the root of who we are has been well documented. Marimba Ani, in her masterwork "Yurugu," and others have discussed the distinction between the basic drives of the European and Afrikan cultures. Afrikans and other people of color, when in our right minds, approach the world in a fundamentally different way from the European. The European cultural asilli[31] and ours are antithetical and mutually exclusive.

We deny who we are and attempt to assume the ethos and culture of our greatest enemies. But we are only dooming ourselves to continued inferiorization and subjugation. We can never be like them, no mater how hard we might try. If we were in our right minds, we would not want to be like them. We can never successfully divorce ourselves from ourselves. We may be able to bleach our skin and hair, but we can never bleach our souls. Tragically, we attempt to fervently, but we only cause deep self-alienation and dissociation. We are by the very nature of our being not white, we are Black — the opposite of white. No matter how hard we try to be like them, we can at best be only white-like. It's kind of like being gold-filled, covered with gold but base metal underneath. We have become whitenized.

So profound is this alienation from ourselves, that among many of us, being called a Black Afrikan is the worst insult that can be hurled at us. Better off talking about someone's mother than to call him or her a Black Afrikan. Folks have killed over words like that.

But call me a Black Afrikan and I will thank you for the compliment. Black Afrikan, in my mind, is the best thing you could call me.

In our self-denial and whitenization, we dissociate ourselves from that which is most valuable and sacred to us — our ancestors. Many Black people have done all they can to erase their family history — the "blackness" is too shameful and hard to bear. It is as if we had enslaved ourselves. We often do not want to know about our past.

Our ancestors want us to reclaim that which is ours. They want nothing more than to see us reclaim the beauty and harmony of The Way, our way,[32] that has been stripped from us. They are working full time to help us open our eyes and see the truth of our own way of life. They are working full time to send us cues, give us intuitions, put others in our path, to help us to reclaim the power and beauty that is ours. When we begin to fully cooperate with our Ori,[33] we will find that Elegba[34] will open all doors for us. We will come into our perfect health driven by spirit, a spirit in need of warriors to restore Maat for our people. We must engage in the process of going back to move forward — Sankofa.[35] We must re-Afrikanize. We must — through active study, spiritual work and self-inquiry — reclaim the root of ourselves, our Afrikanity.

Amos Wilson, Kobi K.K. Kambon, Mwalimu Baruti and other scholar/writers clearly show us that what Wilson termed "the falsification of Afrikan consciousness" and Kambon terms "cultural misorientation"[36] is the root cause of mental illness among Afrikan people. (generational nutricide[37] is another.) It makes sense; if you are thinking and acting like your oppressor/conqueror/enslaver, who by definition has no respect for you, then you will naturally function self-disrespectfully. You will tend operate in a fundamental way alienated from, and disrespectful of yourself because you have accepted the thought patterns and cultural trappings of those who have exploited your ancestors and continue to exploit you.

How then can one be expected to take good care of oneself? As stated earlier, the most important aspect of health is self-awareness. It is the ability to clearly perceive what is going on inside and around you. It is the ability to accurately interpret the subtle signs God is giving you through your sensations, intuitions and dreams. If you are thinking as your enemy does, how can you do anything other than misinterpret those thoughts and come to conclusions that are against your own best interest?

If I am alienated from myself, how can I correctly perceive what those subtle messages are saying? If I deny the beauty, primacy and righteousness of my existence by using a foreign thought pattern and belief system, how then can I correctly think through and apply the knowledge I gain? How can I accurately perceive and respond to the messages I receive from my environment and from God if I am functioning in a mindset that is diametrically opposed to the health of my people and to me as a individual?

We must regain our right minds if we are to be able to effectively heal any disease. More than any other factor, the falsification of our consciousness is at the root, and unless we address it, it will prevent the healing of the diseases of our people.

Afrikan people know there is no separation of us from our families and communities. Our traditional focus has been on the collective first. Our primordial Afrikan though process was because we are — I am. Afrikan traditional cultural institutions made sure the No. 1 priority is the health of the family and community. If in our colonized state of mind we are thinking with an individualistic (read eurocentric) mind, then how can we see to it that the Afrikan community is healthy?

Frances Cress Welsing says that nothing else will make sense until we understand racism/white supremacy. Until we understand the system that continues to oppress us, we will be unable to properly interpret our senses, sensations, intuitions, dreams and the events around us because — we will do it from the mindset of those who would oppress us. We can only be confused as to what our own best interest is.

In the final analysis, we cannot be fully aware and we cannot be fully healthy until we are in our right minds.

We must go back and fetch our conscious minds as Afrikan people in order to throw off this mesmeric[38] state that has rendered us unable to effectively seek and find solutions to our problems. We must shed the veil that has us unable to effectively interpret our intuitions and sensations that the Divine continuously provides us to guide our lives. We must re-learn to love our natural Afrikan selves that we may sincerely focus on our health and the health of our communities. We must truly love ourselves that we may generate consistent positive self-talk and action. We must love ourselves to love others.

15. We Must Have A Habitual Practice Of Loving Kindness

Love heals all. Giving loving kindness to others and the expression of affection are the most wonderful and healing sensations/experiences known. At our fundamental core we are love. We are born with few abilities that manifest in infancy. One of these is the ability to love. Infants are love machines. They have the ability to give love radiantly to those who engage them. If not suppressed, this quality will continue throughout life. It is this ability to give love that makes our lives worth living. I thank my wife regularly for being so lovable and so receptive to my love. When I express my love for others, I feel peace, calmness and warmth of spirit. Whatever might be bothering me quickly fades. I have no doubt it is the best thing in life.

Second best is receiving unconditional love from others. Approval and acknowledgement are balms to the soul. Many of us lack this in sufficient quantities. Many of us have been hurt by insincere compliments and fake adoration and are unable to receive that affection. Despite having someone who truly loves and shows affection, some of us cannot receive it because of the wounds on our soul. This is why giving false affection/acknowledgement for the purpose of seduction is one of the worst things you can do. In the superficial, predatory culture in which we live, this is often the curse of those most physically or socially attractive. They experience so much empty or self-serving praise that they come to doubt any praise they receive. They paradoxically come to feel they are not truly lovable because they see so much "love" for their persona, that they trust no one.

One of the most beautiful things about giving love is that love tends to cycle back to you. It may not be requited from the person you give it to, but it invariably comes back in one way or another. You can never run out of love that you give freely and without conditions. My advice is for you to find people to love, people who are able to genuinely receive your love, and freely, without restraint, give them all the love you have. Odds are they are the people who will most likely be able to cycle it back to you.

16. We Must Engage In Right Livelihood

One of the problems with modern life in the West and increasingly throughout the rest of the world is the notion that we can separate what we do from who we are. It is commonplace to say, "I am not my job," or "That's just what I do for a living; it's not who I am." We believe that if in our off time we are good people, then that is all that matters. Many of us have come to believe we can do wrong or even outright evil things at work, and dismiss this as something we had to do to feed our family. We either deny the truth or rationalize and excuse ourselves as we do work that has negative effects on the world. We trick ourselves into believing we have no responsibility for the poisoned fruit of our labor. We rationalize that we are only a small part of the "Evil Empire" and that we did not start it and in fact are secretly opposed to the product or service it produces.

Deep down inside, if only on a subconscious level, we know that we reap what we sow. If you are playing tug-of-war and your team wins, no matter how hard you did or didn't pull, you get credit for the win. When you show up at work, you are stating that this is what my life force is contributing to. This is what my attention and energy is devoted to. Then we go and say it doesn't count when the final tally is made. We believe the legal definition of corporation is a person and thus this paper entity is the culprit, not we who actually do the deeds.

I'm saying to you right now that is does matter. When Judgment Day comes, all our actions will be counted. Doing things just for the money doesn't exempt us from the bad karma[39] that we generate. Good is rewarded with good and evil is rewarded with evil no matter what time of day it is done. And what is money, anyway? Money is only a form of energy. It is merely a tool for trade. It is true that the sins of the father are visited upon the son. This can mean that the children learn to sin by watching their parents, or it can mean that misfortune is due to the child of those who sin. Or it can mean that in future lifetimes, suffering will result from evil caused in this life.

To live in true abundance, we must come to learn that we have a purpose, and that God and our ancestors are in league with us to fulfill this purpose. We cannot succumb to a mentality of lack, believing that to survive we must compromise our values and do something that is not in alignment with righteousness. We must have faith that we are supposed to live our purpose and work in right livelihood for good. If we do so, the Divine will abundantly provide for our needs. When we are in right livelihood, all that we need appears before us on the road of life. *A healthy life is one where there is congruency and consistency with Maat in all that we do.* We have to believe that God and our ancestors reward doing the right thing now.

Affirmation: *Regardless of appearances, we are whole, perfect and complete. We have everything we need to heal all matter of illness, disease or injury in us right now. We have always had it in us. We do not need anyone else to heal us. We respect and follow our ancestral wisdom as it guides us on our path.*

Acid Vs. Alkaline?

Patients frequently ask about special water or supplements to alkalinize the system, so a brief mention is in line.

False belief: my body is out of whack with acid, and I need to correct this with a supplement, special water or a drug. I need to eat loads of protein to maintain my strength, vitality and virility.

PH is the measure of the relative amount of acid and alkaline in a chemical mix. The lower the pH, the more acid the substance is. For example, hydrochloric acid has a very low pH of 1.1. Sodium hydroxide (lye) has a very high pH of 12.9. Pure water is a neutral pH 7.0. The body guards its acid-base balance carefully so that all of the pH-dependent biochemical reactions take place normally. The blood is kept by the body at very close to a slightly alkaline 7.4. An alteration of 0.3-0.5 in the pH of the blood in either direction is very severe and often fatal. The body has very powerful mechanisms to maintain that balance, at almost any cost.

Buffering

A buffer is a chemical which when mixed with other chemicals will tend to stabilize or resist change in the pH of a liquid. We know the body must maintain tight control over its pH. The principal organs involved in the buffering of the bloodstream are the lungs, kidneys and bones. The lungs adjust the amount of carbon dioxide in the bloodstream. The bones help buffer by leaching calcium and phosphorus into the bloodstream, when an excessive acid load is present. The kidneys excrete this calcium/phosphorus/acid load into the urine. (The kidneys also have other mechanisms as well for maintaining the balance, which I won't elaborate on here.)

Acid Ash vs. Alkaline Ash

The residue left over after a food or other substance is metabolized or burned is either acidic or alkaline. Dietitians use the term acid ash or alkaline ash to classify foods, because historically foods were burned and the leftover "ash" residue was tested for pH. High-protein foods such as red meat, poultry, dairy products, fish, shellfish and eggs are acidic in residue. Alcohol, although it is not acid ash, is metabolized to acid. Vegetable foods with few exceptions become alkaline ash. When a person eats excess protein or excess fats that their body cannot use in its daily metabolism, the liver metabolizes it. These products are stored as body fat, and the remaining waste products are acidic and must be cleared from the bloodstream.

The same is true for any amount of alcohol. This clearing is done primarily by the kidneys, and is excreted into the urine. But before these acidic-breakdown products can be removed from the bloodstream, the body must protect itself from changes in pH by neutralizing/buffering the acid.

One of the ways this acid is neutralized is by buffering it with calcium and phosphorus in various forms. The kidney then must excrete the entire complex, leading to calcium loss if excessive amounts of acid-forming foods (protein and fat) are consumed. It should come as no surprise that low protein diets are used routinely to treat patients with liver and kidney failure. Certain parts of the body, such as the stomach and vagina, are naturally maintained as an acid environment. The acidity in these areas kills or inhibits certain microorganisms. This mechanism occurs naturally and maintains the balance throughout the body. Not so with an excessive intake of acid-forming foods.

What Are The Consequences?

The direct consequences of an acid-forming diet include: arthritis, kidney stones and kidney failure, osteoporosis, inflammation and pain. There are multitudes of consequences of eating an animal-based diet, which have been well documented.

High-protein diets cause serious metabolic changes that lead to bone loss and kidney stones. The acid load from high-protein animal foods must be buffered. As I mentioned earlier, the bones supply the calcium and phosphorus to accomplish this. This calcium and phosphorus passes into the urine and often forms kidney stones when water intake is inadequate. An acid-forming diet also enhances and augments cravings for alkaline-based drugs such as caffeine, cocaine (crack), heroin, nicotine, amphetamine and cannabis. A person who is attempting to withdraw from these addictive drugs should alkalinize their bloodstream.

So, What's The Bottom Line?

To maintain balance and stave off drug cravings, arthritis, kidney stones and kidney failure, osteoporosis, inflammation and a variety of other problems, respect your natural diet. Respect your body and it will work just fine. Avoid an excessive acid load in the form of high-protein intake. Do not confuse your body's natural appetites by taking in alkaline drugs (including certain prescription medications). Milk is not a good calcium source because it is high in protein; the acid load overbalances the calcium. No surprise, regions that have the highest milk intake also experience a high rate of osteoporosis.

High protein foods such as red meat, poultry, fish, shellfish, dairy and eggs, all of which metabolize to acid, should also be avoided to maintain the body's acid/alkaline balance.

Consume only modest amounts of vegetable protein — vegans are not immune to this problem.

Drink lots of water, which enhances kidney function.

Avoid alkaloid drugs, such as caffeine and nicotine, which stimulate the craving for acid-producing foods.

Eat a diet that is high in alkaline-forming foods, such as fresh fruit and vegetables.

Avoid alcohol.

Dietary supplements cannot and should not take the place of proper diet and in general should be avoided. Eat well and smart instead.

Affirmation: *My body is in perfect balance. I naturally desire and take into my system that which is good, nourishing and health promoting. I have everything I need to heal anything within me right now.*

Have You Got The Teeth For Beef?

The best of mankind is a farmer; the best food is fruit. — Ethiopia

Patients sometimes tell me that a vegetarian diet leaves them weak, cold and lacking in energy. They report that after they put meat back into their diets they felt stronger and warmer. What's up with that?

False Belief: We need to eat flesh to stay strong and vibrant. We need external tools to prepare and eat our food.

If You Cain't Eat It Raw — Just Say Naw!

Animals are distinct from plants and microorganisms as they must consume other living things to survive. With few exceptions, all animals eat their food fresh and alive whenever possible. No animal has the need to refrigerate, incinerate, scald, poach, sauté, bake, braise or otherwise heat or alter with bacteria or chemicals its food to render it safe for consumption. Like other animals, the human body was designed to eat its food raw. I know some people have a hard time seeing us as animals despite their own sometimes "animalistic" behavior, but why would we be designed any differently than other living creatures? What godly or evolutionary advantage would such a design meet? Therefore, any food we cannot safely eat raw is not necessary for good health and can be avoided.

Eat What You Are Supposed To Eat, Where You Are Supposed To Live

Just as with the so-called lower animals, our bodies are designed perfectly. Our hands, feet, eyes, musculature, skin, genitals and digestive tracts are perfectly designed for their function. Homo sapiens are the most adaptable animal species, and that has allowed us to survive far outside of our natural habitats, which are regions where we can comfortably exist without clothing. Those areas are tropical and forested and provide warmth and shade for our predominantly hairless bodies. In these regions, all the food we need is naturally abundant. However, because we can adapt to other areas, it does not mean we will thrive there. Many of our modern dis-ease states are a direct consequence of living in areas in which we were not designed to live.

Form Follows Function

All species of animals have efficient, built-in equipment that allows consumption and digestion of food and elimination of waste. The mouth, teeth, stomach, pancreas, liver and intestinal tract are custom designed for processing food. The stomach juices of carnivorous animals have a very high concentration of acid and digestive enzymes that break down proteins and fats. The high level of acid is needed to sterilize the enormous amount of microorganisms in the food they consume. Typically, carnivores will eat the intestines and other internal organs of their prey first, because to them it is the delicacy. The feces inside the intestines are loaded with bacteria that would make even the carnivorous animal sick if the high acid in their stomach did not kill the bacteria. As natural vegetarians (herbivores), our stomachs do not have the capability of creating the very high level of acid of carnivores. This is why we must first kill and render relatively sterile the bacteria-laden meat. We do this by heating or processing it (sushi eaters are welcome to submit their argument here). And because we are adaptable, we can ramp up our acid production to tolerate the high fat/protein load in the form of meat. Consequently, we find peptic ulcer disease, esophagitis — and the vast majority of other health problems related to eating flesh — are increasing in epidemic proportions.

Ask Your Dentist: If You Ain't Got The Teeth — Don't Mess With Beef!

The hands/paws, claws, talons and teeth that animals have are designed to manipulate the food they eat. Animals that eat certain types of foods have similar equipment to that of other types of animals eating the same type of foods. Carnivorous animals have sharp, pointed teeth that allow them to grasp and kill prey and rip flesh from the bone, which they crush and swallow with minimal chewing. Human are poorly equipped for this. Our hands, teeth and digestive tract are designed to consume fruits, vegetables, nuts, sprouted grains and sprouted legumes.

If You Are Feeling Cold, Move To A Warmer Climate

All animals have a natural range or habitat. Only people and cockroaches live all over the world. Perhaps if it weren't for our extreme adaptability and intellect, we would use our instinctual wisdom to accept our abundance, refuse to believe in lack and consume only that which our ancestors knew to be natural. Had we not migrated to areas that are inhospitable to our bodies, and remained where it was comfortable to live without having to light fires, weave cloth and wear the skin of animals, we might have kept eating the foods that grew in the areas where we naturally lived. I know we are not all going to pick up and move to the tropics. That does not mean you can violate the principles that all animals live by: Eat food raw and in season in the areas to which we are naturally indigenous.

But Nana Kwaku - I'm Still Feeling Cold

Some people who go on a vegan diet feel weak and cold because they are not eating a balance of the right kinds of foods for their body type, within the wide variety of plant food available. If you indulge in fad diets or processed foods and do not wisely balance warm/cooling foods, yin/yang foods, spicy, sweet, salty, sour and pungent foods, do not be surprised if you are not feeling up to snuff. If you feel cold, you can eat a heavier, warmer diet. Consuming a heavy, hot, spicy meal can make you feel warmer. This can be accomplished easily and effectively with information about the nature of foods and spices without having to resort to eating flesh. If millions of Hindus and Buddhists living in a variety of climates can thrive without eating flesh, so can you. Eat mindfully. Re-learn to follow your appetite very carefully.

Listen to your body. Pay close attention to how you feel physically, mentally, emotionally and spiritually, before and after you eat. Eat whole, fresh and unadulterated foods. Trust your instinct and you will naturally make good, sound food choices.

Affirmation: *The natural world abundantly provides me with all that I need for vibrant health and energy. I understand and follow natural laws that apply to all sentient beings.*

How Now Mad Cow

In 2004, the news of a lone infected cow in Washington State hit the mass media like a freight train. Other infections were found, but there has been very little in the press since then, effectively blacking out a very important and haunting story that has profound implications for everyone who eats animal products. What is the real deal about this, and should you concern yourself with it?

False belief: Animals are chemical factories for protein. It matters not what we feed them nor are there any consequences to human health for forcing the animals into an unnatural diet and consuming them as food.

It is now well accepted that people can get the fatal brain disorder, also known as mad cow disease, also known as spongiform encephalopathy or variant Creutzfeldt-Jakob disease (CJD), from eating infected beef. What is not well known is that the animal does not have to be sick to pass it on. All tests so far indicate that if an animal is fed the infected remains of another animal, it also becomes contaminated. In other words, it is possible to contract this disease from eating any animal product!

Prions For Animal Peons

The infectious agent that causes this scourge is called a prion. Prions are not themselves alive and contain no DNA. In fact, prions are abnormally shaped versions of a protein that is found in all animal tissues and blood. They are not found in plants. These proteins are quite durable and are not destroyed by any routine disinfecting technique. Cooking has no effect on them. These prions are transmitted from any animal to any other animal by ingestion of flesh or body fluids. It is not yet known how many prions one must consume to induce the disease. Gradually, more of the normal-shaped proteins metamorph into the deformed, abnormally shaped proteins by a process not yet well understood. In large enough concentration, these prions wreak havoc on the brain. Until then, it incubates stealthily. In modern industrial ranching, the animals live a fraction of their normal life span and are slaughtered before disease manifests symptomatically. They don't live long enough to get sick and thereby get culled from the herd. Yet, ominously these animals can still transmit CJD.

Road-Kill Fed Beef, Vampire Veal, Cannibal Cows, With Feces Eating Grins? Or, Is That Poor Fido Mixed Into That Feed?

In modern industrial farming, little raw material is wasted. The rendering industry takes animal waste, processes it and sells it back to the ranchers in the form of feed products for the animals. Included in this "protein concentrate" is waste of every kind of dead animal, chicken feces, pig feces, road kill and dog pound remains. Even veterinary-euthanized animals are collected, ground up, cooked and turned into animal feed. In North America, calves are literally weaned on milk formula containing "raw spray-dried cattle blood plasma," even though scientists have known for many years that blood can transmit mad cow-type diseases. In addition to cattle blood being fed back to cattle, billions of pounds of fat, blood meal, meat and bone meal from pigs and poultry are also rendered and fed to cattle. In turn, cattle are rendered and fed to other species, a perfect environment for spreading and amplifying mad cow disease and even for creating new strains of the disease.[40]

Michael Hansen, a scientist for Consumers Union, points out that cattle tissues that are mostly removed from the human food chain are still converted to feed for chickens, pigs and fish, among others. And remains of those animals are again rendered into cattle feed — a practice denounced by critics and banned in Europe but still legal and commonplace in the United States. "Those animals could become silent carriers and infect cattle," Hansen says.

Cattle Are Ruminants And Don't Need To Eat Protein

Cattle have practically zero dietary requirements for protein. All species of animals have efficient, built-in equipment to allow them to gather, consume, digest and eliminate food and waste. The mouth, teeth, stomach, pancreas, liver, and intestinal tract are designed for processing food that is readily available in the habitat in which the animal is most comfortable. In basic zoology, we learned that cattle and horses are ruminants. Ruminants have several stomachs that contain huge amounts of bacteria that turn grass and air into proteins. Cattle are perfectly designed to eat grass and leaves. They derive all of their nutrients from this. Feeding ruminants a protein concentrate from animal remains has no functional purpose other than more profits for the flesh-exploiting industry. Forcing naturally herbivorous animals into becoming cannibals, vampires, and feces-eaters is draconian, execrable, vile, utterly repugnant and morally reprehensible. It is as horrible and wrong as murder or chattel slavery.

Doc, Are You Sure Grandma Has Alzheimer's?

Over recent decades, the rates of Alzheimer's disease in the United States have skyrocketed. According to the Centers for Disease Control, Alzheimer's is now the eighth leading cause of death, afflicting an estimated 4 million Americans. But 20 percent or more of people clinically diagnosed with Alzheimer's disease are found at autopsy not to have had Alzheimer's at all. A number of autopsy studies have shown that a small percentage of Alzheimer's deaths may in fact be CJD. Given the new research showing that infected beef may be responsible for some sporadic CJD, thousands of Americans may already be dying because of mad cow disease every year.

Prion disease expert Carlton Gajdusek, for example, estimates that 1 percent of patients visiting Alzheimer's clinics actually have CJD. In a Yale study, of 46 patients clinically diagnosed with Alzheimer's, six were proven to have CJD at autopsy. In another study of brain biopsies, of a dozen patients diagnosed with Alzheimer's, three of them were actually dying from CJD. An informal survey of neuropathologists registered a suspicion that CJD accounts for 2 to 12 percent of all dementias. Two autopsy studies showed a CJD rate among dementia deaths of about 3 percent. A third study, at the University of Pennsylvania, showed that 5 percent of patients diagnosed with dementia had CJD. Although only a few hundred cases of sporadic CJD are officially reported in the U.S. annually, hundreds of thousands of Americans die with dementia every year. Thousands of these deaths may actually be from CJD caused by eating infected meat.[41]

Russian Roulette At The Dinner Table Anyone?

We can now be certain that there is a finite risk of contracting CJD from eating virtually any animal product. But what is the risk? The answer is we don't exactly know, and won't know until it is too late to do anything for those who have taken an "it can't harm me" attitude.

Suppose you had a revolver with 100,000 chambers in it pointed at your temple. Every time you eat animal products, you squeeze the trigger. Only you don't know how many bullets are in the gun. Are you feeling lucky? Have another bite of that chili cheeseburger and make your day.

Humans Are Natural Vegans And Don't Need To Eat Any Animals

The lower animals that people eat for food are not "lower" at all, but are beings with feelings. How do we resolve the fact that the animals we eat have memories, babies, feel pain, and suffer? Can we call ourselves civilized or humane if we insatiably exploit without reason?

The fact remains unequivocally we shouldn't be eating animals in the first place. We can live our lives in accordance with natural law that firmly and without doubt places us as vegetarians. We can eat well, feel great, and never ever taste any animal products. This is accomplished easily and effectively with some simple information about the nature of foods and spices without ever having to resort to eating flesh or animal body fluids.

You can get everything you need to be healthy and vibrant from your food, just as other herbivorous animals do, without resorting to the survival tactic of consuming other animals or their vital fluids. (See "Have You Got The Teeth For Beef?") There is no biological requirement for human beings to eat any animal product for optimal health. So, why would we take the risk of our brain turning to sponge just for the taste or "satisfaction" of eating flesh?

We Are All Addicts!

The vast majority of health problems people suffer from are a consequence of their addictions. As a physician who is directed by spirit to help my people heal, I have come to the realization that is it is nearly impossible to address the majority of chronic health problems without addressing addiction and at its root, the falsification of our consciousness/cultural misorientation.

Addiction — What Is It?

Behavior

All addictions involve a self-destructive behavior of some sort. This behavior is experienced as pleasurable, at least at first.

Repetitive

This behavior is done over and over again.

Out Of Control

The addicted person, although they usually believe to the contrary, has no effective control on limiting how much or how often the behavior is conducted to avoid adverse consequences.

Harmful

The addictive behavior is either directly or indirectly harmful to the addict.

Denial

The addict has little or no conscious awareness that they have an addictive pattern of behavior and when confronted will deny a problem exists.

Tolerance

Increasing frequency or amounts of the behavior must be done to achieve the pleasurable state.

Dependency

The person is compelled by the addiction to engage in the behavior to feel normal. Without the behavior the person feels abnormal and dysphoric. Ultimately, the person will perform the behavior to merely feel normal; to not feel sick.

Withdrawal

Upon discontinuation of the behavior, the person experiences often-intense physical, mental, emotional, psychic symptoms that are extinguished only by resuming the behavior. This sensation will last throughout a period of detoxification until the addict's system has completely — if only temporarily — purged the behavior.

Craving

When not performing the behavior the addict will have often unbearably intense craving desires to engage in the behavior, sometimes completely consuming his conscious awareness.

Periods Of Abstinence

The addict will "clean up" at times and not engage in the behavior, yet the addiction persists and the craving may continue to varying degrees.

Relapse

The addict will periodically resume the addictive behavior often more intensely. The phenomenon of relapse has several stages involving mental, emotional, spiritual and psychic processes that occur predictably before the addict actually resumes the behavior. Addiction counseling focuses on bringing to awareness the stages of relapse and seeks to empower the addict to interrupt the process as early as possible with techniques that have predictably prevented the behavior in the past.

Addiction Is Fundamentally Both Caused By And Is A Response To A Separation From Spirit

In Afrikan cosmology, just before our people are incarnated, we come to this life with an agreement with the spirit world. That agreement is made in concert with our ancestors, with our guiding deities and with God. We agree that there is a path that we are to take and we come to life having embodied the soul essence of one of our ancestors who had transitioned to the spirit realm and who is dedicated to that path. Sometimes the individual is born of spirit itself and is a human manifestation of an aspect of God. The person therefore has aspects of the consciousness that came before him/her. Each of us has a purpose. We each have a role in the advancement and organization of our lineage and our people. We each have a role to play. We each have what the Yoruba call an Ori. The Ori is our "head." It is our guiding mind if you will. It is our spirit purpose in life. The goal of life is to fulfill our Ori. One prays for fulfillment of our Ori, to our Orisha, to our ancestors, and to God. They help us through the spirit world, infusing everything in existence. Spirit and material are inseparable. Our consciousness is the fundamental expression of our soul and is our link to spirit.

Addiction is fundamentally a response to desacralization, a separation from spirit. It is the combination of self-destructive behavior that, paradoxically, temporarily gives the sensation of the soul's craving for connection to the divine. It is a temporary balm that gives the soul the momentary illusion that its soul purposes are being met. Yet when the rush wears off, there is an even deeper hole in our soul because of the delay in its completion of purpose. What in part makes an addictive behavior so compulsive, so beyond our ability to control, is when the behavior is engaged, the soul's purpose is ignored and it is left craving this need to be fulfilled.

Since the spirit/soul is fundamentally affected by addiction, it is essential to treat the addict with a spiritual approach. In European society, this is done through the twelve steps program. It uses a Euro-cosmology appropriate for European people. Because we Afrikans have our own cosmology and spiritual tradition, we should use our own spiritual traditions in the treatment of addiction. The twelve steps program is non-secular but based the cosmology of the Caucasian.

Cultural misorientation is the root cause of all of our health problems. That Afrikan people exist under a system of mental enslavement is understood and will not be argued here. Key to enslavement and colonization of a people is the falsification of their consciousness — the elimination of original consciousness and the imposition of the cultural consciousness of the enslaver/colonizer. Our enslavement is maintained by the falsification of our Afrikan consciousness, and imposition of an alien mindset. We have been forcibly separated from our native cosmology and spiritual tradition. The imposition of a foreign religion and cosmology and ultimately culture is key to domination and control of a people and it has always been imposed by invaders/enslavers.

When the soul suffers from a falsified conscious state, it struggles to regain its natural consciousness. Its Nananom/Egungun and Abossom/Orisha help it on a subconscious level. However, addiction tends to maintain the separation that leaves a hole in the spirit. That separation is paradoxically temporarily soothed by the addictive behavior. Treatment of addiction, if it is to lead to healing, must first address discontinuation of that destructive behavior and then reconnection with our original Afrikan consciousness.

Imposition of addiction and foreign religion are always used in an attempt to colonize and enslave. As long as we allow ourselves to function with a foreign mindset and engage in addictive behaviors, we will be enslaved. As long as we function from a foreign-imposed mindset, we will be unhealthy.

Clinically, I see a trend where the patients who have the greatest degree of their Afrikan consciousness intact are the most successful in healing their addiction and their medical problems. The process of addiction treatment in people of Afrikan descent therefore must include re-verification of their Afrikan self-consciousness.

Freeing yourself from addiction is a revolutionary act because it opens your soul to connecting with itself. An addiction-free person is much better able to pursue fulfillment of their Ori — the mission you were born to fulfill. As we struggle with foreign domination of our land, economies and minds, it is natural that our Ori is directed towards liberation. Using drugs and other harmful substances or engaging in other addictive acts is counterrevolutionary. If you come across a person or group that calls itself revolutionary but has a culture of drug use or SAD (standard American diet), they are in fact counterrevolutionary despite their rhetoric. Soul food destroys the soul. Their behavior reinforces their own addiction and mental enslavement. It leads to illness and early death. If Afrikan people are to be free from this system of white supremacy, we must get this point.

The war on drugs declared in the 1980s was in fact a war — using drugs — on people of color, especially Afrikan people. Crack cocaine was brought into our communities, our people became addicted to it and then were criminalized for their weakness. A new Jim Crow has been placed on our people based on the legalized discrimination against convicted felons.[42] This has entrenched the economic enslavement of our people and reinforced the mental enslavement.

Metabolic syndrome, with its deadly constellation of diabetes, obesity, hypertension, hyperlipidemia and atherosclerotic vascular disease, is the new scourge of our people. These diseases have become pandemic among us, offshoots of our addictive illnesses. Addictive use of animal products and food-like substances is the cause of this problem. The treatment and prevention are the same. Withdrawal and recovery from addiction to animal products, sugar and other food-like substances are without doubt the path to the healing of metabolic syndrome.

A huge part of economy is based on the addictive consumption of addictive food products that cause illness. The animal husbandry, agricultural, food processing, advertising, grocery, automotive/trucking /rail, chemical, oil, pharmaceutical, fast food, hospital, medical technology, medical laboratory, environmental, and health insurance industries would suffer a major blow and might even collapse if people stopped poisoning themselves with these products. Freeing yourself from the grip of addiction to drugs, animal products and cooked foods is perhaps the most revolutionary act you can do, as well as the most environmentally positive. While it is not possible by itself to eat your way to health, eating properly is a powerful act toward maximal health.

When all of existence is viewed as sacred, when all behavior is seen as part of divine order, when living in alignment with the natural world where everything is viewed as a part of God, and as incarnate beings, it is our duty to live as spiritual beings manifesting a unique expression in this, the physical realm of Oludumare.[43] When I am in conscious union with the divine, it is difficult if not impossible to contemplate acts that violate our sacred covenant. Only when we mentally separate ourselves from spirit can we accept behavior that is destructive to our physical being. Only when we are removed from spirit can we conceive of voluntarily cooperating with those who would exploit our people or land. Only then can we perceive personal benefit as separate from that of our people.

Yes, of course, many of us will naively blunder into addictive behavior. It is very difficult to become aware that you are in an addictive behavior pattern when everyone you know is also addicted. Because few of us are aware we are addicts we must be gentle with ourselves and with others.

I am convinced that the act of re-Afrikanization and its attendant re-sacralization is the most important thing we can do to awaken ourselves to our addictive patterns.

What Is This Process Of Re-Afrikanization?

Re-Afrikanization is the process of reclaiming the common cultural, political, economic, social and spiritual characteristics that are indigenous to

Afrikans. It is the process of learning to discern the distinctions between the culture, behavior and thought patterns of the Afrikan mind compared to those of other cultures. It is the process of accepting the Afrikan mindset as the only appropriate viewpoint for Afrikan people throughout the diaspora. It is the rejection of the concept of a universal mind shared by all people. It is understanding the diametric opposition of the European mindset to that of the Afrikan. It is embracing an Afrikan mindset that is normative, natural and essential for our survival and growth as a people.

Affirmation: Re-Afrikanization is a process of unlearning and learning anew. I shed all aspects of imposed thinking and acculturation that negate my being as an Afrikan and that continues my mental enslavement. I embrace and incorporate Afrikan cultural attributes, behaviors and thought patterns that are good and rightfully mine as a person of Afrikan descent.

What Is The Matrix?

Any race that accepts the thoughts of another race, automatically, becomes the slave race of that other race. — Marcus Mosiah Garvey

The Matrix Is A Prison For Your Mind

The matrix is a prison for your mind. The matrix is the delusionary state of mind created by long-term multi-generational mis-education and propaganda, through which thought and opinion are controlled. The matrix is a major and powerful tool of the system of advanced global monopoly capital and racism/white supremacy. It imposes the state of mental enslavement of which most Afrikans suffer. While in the matrix, the person believes he is operating in free will yet his thoughts, feelings and behavior are manipulated and controlled by the owners of the matrix. Knowledge of the existence of the matrix by its authors has always been most vigorously denied and actively repressed. People who are in the matrix have no perception that they exist in an artificially created state of mind designed for their enslavement. As such, victims of the matrix will vigorously and actively deny its very existence.

The Matrix Tells Us What To Think About And Gives Us The Information That It Wants Us To Use In Forming Our Thoughts

The matrix is what gets us to go to work for oppressive jobs and bosses for ridiculously paltry remuneration. The matrix is what causes us to consistently be unable to unify and work for our own best interests. It causes us to consistently make inappropriate responses to our environment. It leads us to passivity and reactivity, unable to form a proactive thrust to solving our problems. The matrix is the primary mechanism for enforcing the class and race nature of society and maintaining a slave mentality among the former chattel. The matrix is the primary tool for the maintenance of a long-term state of white supremacy.

The Matrix Serves To Separate Us From Ourselves

The matrix maintains us in a thought/mind state that is contrary to our own ascilic drive[44]. It creates and maintains cultural misorientation in which those in the matrix are molded into a cultural formation that is the creation of the architects of the matrix. The matrix is designed to keep us thinking about separation, violence, domination, materialism, linearity, negativity, judgment, time, guilt, blame, greed, individualism, disease and fear, fear, fear. It is dedicated to keeping us from thinking with unity consciousness. It is designed to break our ability to come into conscious union with God, our Nananom, Egungun[45] and our Abossom/Orisha/Loa.[46] It is designed to make us forget that we are not limited to this time and space, and that we are, figuratively and literally, our ancestors and our descendants.

The Afrikan in the matrix typically believes, thinks and holds opinions that have no basis in reality and are invariably antithetical to his own well-being. Most of us were born into the matrix and have no idea anything other than the matrix might exist. If confronted with the reality of the matrix, we will actively rebel, attempt to censure or even kill the bearer of the news.

Many of us live our entire lives with the intermittent, vague, uncomfortable feeling that something is wrong, that the world as we know it is not real. Every now and then, holes in the matrix form and glimpses of the true world are visible to those of us jacked in. Our Nananom and our Abossom/Orisha/Loa who are fighting tirelessly to take back our minds, punch these holes that we may see the truth. Those of us who are disposed to waking up catch fleeting glimpses of our truth before they are expertly wiped over by the designers of the matrix. Often, it is we ourselves who wipe out the light, so conditioned are we to darkness. It is this vague feeling of unease, this subconscious cognitive dissonance that we experience that in part drives us to the addictive use of drugs, junk food and food-like substances, engage in casual or deviant sex, and seek exotic forms of rituals and ceremonies. These distractions momentarily shift us out of a vaguely uncomfortable but all-too-familiar state of delusion.

The matrix is the most tightly held system of false consciousness. The matrix is the post-industrial form of chattel slavery — mental slavery. The purpose of the matrix is to keep us from realizing the truth of our existence in a post-industrial, advanced, white supremacist, monopoly capitalist society — we are enslaved. The matrix is the falsification of our Afrikan consciousness; it is cultural misorientation;[47] it is the yurugu virus. It is highly infectious, and if not carefully and actively offset with truth, our ways and rituals, it can strike, taking over our minds at any time. It is the underlying condition that leads us to mentacide,[48] nutricide, homicide and suicide. It is perhaps the fundamental underlying cause of all disease — mental, emotional, physical and spiritual among Afrikan people.

Principal Characteristics Of The Matrix (adapted from Amos Wilson)*

- Desacralization

- Amnesia

- Pathological Anxiety

- Active Multiple Addictions

- Delusion

- Apathy

- Denial

- Alienation

*These include and are an expansion of the common symptoms of pathological normalcy in oppressed Afrikans, as exposed in "The Falsification Of Afrikan Consciousness" by Amos Wilson, 1993, World Infosystems.

Desacralization

In the matrix, connection with and access to the spirit world is dysfunctional. Our ability to access our traditions that allow us to commune with our ancestors/Nananom/Egungun or patron deities is effectively nullified. This is a central goal of the matrix. The European in his devolution has come to lack a conscious union with the divine. In his earliest dealings with us he became aware that the Afrikan saw the sacred in all of creation; in all of existence. The European saw that this unity with God is our greatest strength and the root of our power. He correctly identified this consciousness as the prerequisite of our greatest technology — the greatest technology ever known. This is our Afrikan spiritual technology that gives us the ability to act on this world through the spirit world and through collaboration with Nananom and Abossom. This power transcends time and space. It allows us to effectively act on the past and future. It is backed by the power of God and is in alignment with Maat. If we are in alignment with our Nananom and the Supreme Being, there is nothing that cannot be accomplished. The European also saw that while our spiritually was our greatest strength it could also, with careful manipulation, be turned against us. It can be turned to a generalized religion that acknowledges and celebrates the existence and power of God, while desacralizing all else and indirectly endorsing desacralized behavior.

Amnesia

While in the matrix the individual has little memory of past events outside of his own family circle. The memories of adverse events affecting the individual that have occurred as a result of the matrix are most effectively repressed. This is why oppressed Afrikan people repeatedly fail to learn from their experiences and are doomed to repeat mistakes.

Pathological Anxiety

In addition to dysphoria as a result of actual adverse conditions, while in the matrix the Afrikan suffers from free-floating anxiety that cannot be directly related to any specific event.

Active Multiple Addictions

The desacralized matrix thought and consciousness pattern is at the root of additive behaviors. The matrix actively encourages and promotes addictive behavioral and thought response to dysphoric states of mind. The advertising industry specifically encourages an addictive response because it is simultaneously the best way to rule and to sell. Multiple addictions characterize almost every person in the matrix. There is very little or no awareness of the addictive nature of the emotional, behavioral and thought response engendered by the matrix. The primary and most important addiction is to the matrix signal itself. That signal is the mass media, both print and broadcast, and its postmodern iterations of the World Wide Web, instant messaging, SMS, email, video gaming, etc. Supporting these signals are all institutions of society including schools and universities, the church, military, judiciary, medical system and entertainment.

Delusion

The matrix is a delusional mind-enslaving state that the prisoners/slaves believe does not exist. The matrix actively promotes beliefs and ideas that have no basis in reality. Despite this, those in the grips of the matrix tightly hold on to these false beliefs. "False beliefs held by an individual which are stubbornly retained and defended despite their logical inconsistencies with objective reality and valid evidence to the contrary. Not only do such beliefs persist directly in the face of contradictory evidence, they persist in the face of continuous negative consequences resulting from their being held."[49]

The matrix implants false memories into the mind through the mediums of music and video, combined with drugs, poisonous food-like substances, insomnia and fatigue. Those enslaved to the matrix have nebulous recollections of fictitious video transmitted images that they actually act on and react to as if they were actual events that took place in their lives.

Apathy

Being "plugged into the matrix" engenders apathy. The victims of the matrix do not care to help themselves and usually in fact are unaware that they are in need of help. Those jacked-in to the matrix functionally do not care to make any effort to change what they feel will "not make any difference anyway." Those plugged in fail consistently to accurately perceive what is occurring around them and do not care enough to make any effort to do anything about it.

Denial

Persons in the matrix will deny the matrix exists, even when confronted with incontrovertible evidence of the existence of its enslaving characteristics. The most common response is to dismiss the evidence as a "conspiracy theory," which by definition, because of the widespread and deeply penetrative nature of the matrix in all aspects of society, means the matrix could not possibly exist. The bearer of the news of the existence of the matrix is therefore usually regarded as paranoid, fantastical, off-kilter and likely insane.

Alienation

Individuals "jacked into" the matrix " feel estranged or separated from; indifferent or hostile toward; unfamiliar with; fearful of; withdrawn from; unconnected to; to have lost remembrance or accurate knowledge of and identity with one's true, undistorted self, historical self and culture, and important segments of reality. ...Feelings of aimlessness, normlessness, purposelessness, hopelessness, meaninglessness; of being unmotivated by one's own self-originated needs and values; of being compelled or retarded by unknown, unknowable, but irresistible forces."

What Are The Remedies For This Matrix?

- Identify clearly for yourself the existence of the matrix.

- Educate our own children. As with any disease an ounce of prevention is worth a pound of cure.

- Avoid and/or minimize exposure to the carrier signal — the mass media, especially television and popular music.

- Focus on active re-Afrikanization.

- Adopt Afrikan spiritual practices. Regular connection with spirit is key.

- Build our own businesses.

- Learn and use Afrikan languages.

- Refrain from social contact with Europeans.

- Read Afrikan writers who are about our liberation.

- Avoid drugs of all kinds, including legal drugs such as alcohol, nicotine, caffeine and sugar.

- Care for your body/mind/spirit temple in accordance with the Rule Book and User Guide.

In the West and in the majority of the continent, the war for the resurrection of Afrikan civilization and the destruction of white supremacy can be fought only for the minds of our people. The matrix is the chain that binds and the walls that hold us. It is the primary weapon of our continued repression and control. It has existed in its earliest forms since the earliest Arab-Caucasian invasion of the north of our land. The matrix has been the most important and powerful weapon used to keep our people in bondage. Our efforts must be directed to its final and total destruction. Abibifahodie (Afrikan liberation in Twi). Free the mind to free the land!

Postscript: I came across a book early in my process of re-Afrikanization and awakening and found it eerie to say the least. The European is so arrogant that in his writings he will indirectly admit to the existence of the matrix. See the below quotes.

"Suppose some case of an apparently serious nature is presented to me. Immediately, I might think about life and God; I would realize there is only one life and that is the life of God, [and our Nananom, our Abossom, our people, our descendants] and because it is the only life it must be eternal, must be omnipresent, and that life must be the life of every individual. Therefore nowhere in heaven or on earth [at any time or place] could there be an impaired life, a diseased life, a dead life, a paralyzed life, or a sinful life. Only mesmeric suggestion [the matrix] can testify to error and that can be reversed in the understanding of the one consciousness..."[50]

"All error is hypnotism [the matrix] claiming to operate as your own thinking. As soon as you realize that the error is not in your thinking or in that of your patient, you separate yourself from the suggestion and become free. Recognizing the error, regardless of its form, as universal hypnotism, or mesmeric suggestion, is the release. As long as the error is not recognized as suggestion or imposed hypnotism, you will remain in sin or disease, lack or limitation [enslavement]. Every appearance of sin or disease, lack or death is but hypnotism [the matrix] claiming to act as your thinking. The realization of this truth [and your re-Afrikanization] is your remedy."[51]

Post postscript: If that doesn't "fry your noodle" then consider again how arrogant the Caucasian is that he would create a movie that would outline all of this for us to see as part of the matrix signal itself. Those of you who have seen the popular movie trilogy learned of the recurring strategy used by the owners of the matrix. Recall that in the movies the architects of the matrix know full well that a finite minority of "humanity" will not accept the programing or will throw off their conditioning and if "left unchecked" will create a "systemic anomaly" that will "eventually destroy the matrix." This affects the real life matrix functioning in the world today. The "machines" (Europeans/ whites/ Caucasians) cryptically created "an oracle" and allowed for the rise of "the one." This individual is then identified and elevated by the matrix in a complex subterfuge, giving an illusion that there is actually a revolution brewing. This subterfuge involves "the oracle" and a manipulated, false faith and hope of "change." This "one" will ultimately lead those (who would try to destroy the matrix, while yet still plugged into it) to their own destruction and a disillusioning failure of the revolution. Afterward, "the one" assumes the role of martyr, temporarily destroying "hope" and faith and in the process allowing for the clear identification of those within the matrix who would be predisposed to throw off the programming as well as those sympathizers outside of the matrix who have allied themselves with "the one." These individuals who have hope that "we will overcome some day" are then neutralized by a plethora of methods, restarting a cycle that will allow the "source code" to be reinserted (actually be allowed to remain) into the populous. Thereby, the cycle is restarted, leading to rebirth of a new "one" that follows the same "oracle" and a fresh movement that follows it.

The lesson here is that you cannot destroy the matrix from within, and that anyone currently plugged into the matrix can be used for further entrenching its control over us.

Affirmation: I choose to free my mind from the control of my enemies. I have the free will to think how I choose. I have the ability, the courage and the power to see the world as it truly is. I think, feel and act in ways that are consistent with the best interest of my family, my people and myself. I know as I travel through the real world I am aided and guided by my Egungun/Nananom on a continuing basis. As I walk through this world, all that I need appears before me to fulfill my Ori, my purpose in life. My "A Team" from the spirit realm places it there.

How To Do A Food Journal

Many people are familiar with a diary. A food diary is a record of what the person eats over a period of time. Typically in traditional dietetics a person would write down what how much and when foods and beverages are consumed. This is a basic tool for determining nutrient and caloric intake. However this is limited in bringing about change.

Dr. Opare recommends a food journal that combines food and beverage intake with thoughts, events, feeling states and other observations. This method helps a person understand that how they eat affects the way they feel, and how they feel affects the way they eat. It helps identify addictive behavior in relation to food. It helps identify what foods are beneficial, and assists Dr. Opare in transitioning patients to healthier patterns of food consumption.

Your food journal belongs to you. It is for your use and is a private document. If you want to share it with Dr. Opare, that is fine. He will want to discuss it with you. In either case, please bring it to appointments and classes/groups.

This is how it is done:

- Keep your journal for as long as you can. The more detailed and the longer you keep it, the more it can help you.

- It is best to use a bound journal with lines or quadrille-ruled.

- Make liberal use of space and words. Use as many pages per day as you need.

- Start a new page with each day, and date each page.

- Write down:

- What you eat/drink, including the brand name and how it was prepared
- How much you eat/drink, including size and number of portions
- When you ate/drank it
- How you emotionally felt before and after you ate/drank it
- What you where doing when you ate/drank it
- What your activities/exercise were that day
- What drugs or medications you took that day
- What recreational substances you took that day including tobacco
- How you slept the night before
- How your body felt that day
- How your libido and sexual functioning manifested that day
- Dreams you remember the night before
- Thoughts or ideas you had that day

Remember this is FOR YOU! If you do a partial or incomplete job in doing your journal, you will limit how much can be gotten out of it. If you put all of your sincerity into your journal, it can be a very powerful tool in your claiming the vibrant healthy you that is you!

About The Author

Dr. Nana Kwaku Opare, MD, MPH, Ca is a pioneer in the natural integrative medicine field. He is co-owner and founder of Opare Integrative Health Care, LLC in Atlanta GA, dedicated to the healing of the Afrikan community through medical practice and educational programs in food, nutrition, body movement and spiritual growth. He is a long-term vegan and more recent living food lifestyle practitioner and advocate. He has practiced Eastern and Western Medicine for more than a quarter century.

Nana Kwaku Opare, MD, MPH, CA, BS, graduated from UC Berkely, earning both a BS degree studying Food, Nutrition and Dietetics and a Master's of Public Health degree. He earned his Medical Degree at UC San Francisco and his Certificate in Acupuncture at the San Francisco College of Acupuncture and Oriental Medicine. He trained in Osteopathic Manual Medicine at Michigan State College of Osteopathic Medicine.

Endnotes

---

[1] Yurugu or "the pale fox" originally Ogo is "a being in the Dogon mythology which is responsible for disorder in the universe" and, is the title of the master work written by Marimba Ani, Yurugu, An Afrikan-centered critique of European Cultural Thought and Behavior. (AFDJ, 2009) Here the word is used to describe addiction to the European way of thought and life. It reflects not only a way of thought but also a fundamental cultural drive characteristic of the European and distinctly and fundamentally diametrically opposite of that of Afrikan thought and culture. Therefore if a person of Afrikan origin is to think and behave in a fashion that is consistent with his/her best interests it is essential that they first understand the distinction between Euro and Afrikan thought and culture and orient themselves in alignment with that of the Afrikan original cultural mindset. This is a fundamental and essential concept that the Afrikan person must come to an understanding of on their path to freeing themselves from mental enslavement. This concept will be referred to repeatedly throughout this work.

[2] Cultural Darwinism or Cultural evolution is the concept that cultures evolve as do species. Therefore the latest and the most dominant culture is the best. This doctrine is at the core of the European self-image of superiority of their culture. They are the latest and greatest and thus must be the best and the most deserving and the most correct. The same doctrine extends to all institutions of society including medicine.

[3] K.M Adams, K.C. Lindell, M.K., and S.H. Zeisel, *Status of Nutrition Education in Medical Schools*, American Journal of Clinical Nutrition. 2006 April ; 83(4): 941S–944S.

[4] As a share of GDP, the United States spent 17.4% on health in 2009, 5 percentage points more than in the next two countries, the Netherlands and France (which allocated 12.0% and 11.8% of their GDP on health). Norway and Switzerland were the next biggest spenders on health per capita,

with spending of more than $5000 per capita in 2009. OECD Health Data 2011.

[5] Barbara Starfield, MD, MPH, *Is US Health Really the Best in the World?*, JAMA. 2000; 284(4): 483-485.

[6] The word Nana is a title of honor in the Akan language that priests, priestess, kings, queens, chiefs or queen mothers are given when they are "enstooled" (elevated to the honored position). In my case I was named Nana Kwaku Opare at the Aconedi Shrine at Larteh, Ghana, in honor of the great ancestor priestess, Okomfohemma Nana Akua Oparebea, who transitioned into the ancestral realm months before my first visit to Ghana in 1996. Akomfo means priest or priestess.

[7] Ibid.

[8] Usage of the term *Maafa* was popularized by Professor Marimba Ani's 1994 book <u>Let the Circle Be Unbroken: The Implications of African Spirituality in the Diaspora</u>. (Red Sea Press). Maafa is a Kiswahili term which means great destruction. The term is used to describe the events and experiences of Afrikans at home and throughout the diaspora as a result of the conquest, colonization, and destruction wrought upon us by the Arab and later European invaders/colonizers/enslavers. Also called Afrikan holocaust.

[9] Op.cit.

[10] ● 62.1% of all bankruptcies stem from medical debt.

● Most medical debtors were well educated and middle class; three quarters had health insurance.

● The share of bankruptcies attributable to medical problems rose by percent between 2001 and 2007. *Medical Bankruptcy in the United States, 2007: Results of a National Study,* David U. Himmelstein, MD, Deborah Thorne, PhD, Elizabeth Warren, JD, Steffie Woolhandler, MD, MPH, American Journal of Medicine, 2009.

[11] The US has a death rate ranking 89th in the world of 225, CIA World Fact Book 2011. US death rate is higher than that of Haiti, Eritrea, and more than twice that of the West Bank.

[12] The Physicians' Foundation, The Physicians' Perspective: Medical Practice in 2008; October 2008.

[13] I do think having a policy that will cover you for injuries is probably a good idea. Also it is a lot cheaper to buy than regular health insurance.

[14] See Marimba Ani, Yurugu. This is the essence of European cultural drive and worldview.

[15] Desacralization is the process by which things that are normally construed as sacred are through the force of alien cultural impositions are stripped of their sacred nature. They are no longer considered divine or worthy of reverence. The alienation and objectification of nature. In this view, nature becomes and adversary. This approach to reality originates in unnaturalness.

[16] Ibid.

[17] Isfet is the Kemetic term that refers to chaos, especially worsening chaos. See Kwame Agyei, and Akua Nson Akoto, The Sankofa Movement: ReAfrikanization and the Reality of War (Oyoko InfoCom Inc.; 1st edition 2000).

[18] Khephra is the Kemetic term that is the opposite of Isfet. It is the state of the process of returning to Maat. All that is harmonious and good. See ibid.

[19] See chapter by this name in this book.

[20] Center for Disease Control, *Morbidity and Mortality Weekly Report Supplement,* Vol. 60, January 14, 2011.

[21] See T. Colin Campbell, <u>The China Study</u> (BenBella Books, 2006); Gabriel Cousens, <u>There Is a Cure for Diabetes</u> (North Atlantic Books, 2008); many others.

[22] This concept by Marimba Ani professes that the state of mind of the European=yurugu is infectious and will tend to affect those who come in contact with Europeans behaving like a virus.

[23] A term popularized by Kamau Kambon. Whitenization is the process of personality change that occurs in oppressed Afrikans under conditions of white supremacy as a consequence of that oppression. It is the condition of thinking and behaving as if one where white.

[24] Amos Wilson, <u>The Falsification of Afrikan Consciousness.</u> (Afrikan World Infosystems; 1st edition July 1993). Falsification of consciousness is the process where a person's true native/original consciousness is replaced with a false consciousness of those oppressing him/her.

[25] John Robbins, author of "Diet for a New America."

[26] Mwalimu Baruti, <u>The Sex Imperative</u> (Akoben House). This concept scribes a culturally imposed addictive drive to have sex at all times regardless of the native cultural appropriateness of the behavior.

[27] Maat is the set of Kemetic ethical principles collectively embracing the values of truth, justice, harmony, balance, cosmological order, reciprocity and propriety. Maat is maximal order. Maat is the state of maximal harmony an order in the world.

[28] The zone is a space where things flow with effortless ease.

[29] Manifest Destiny is a concept of white supremacist thought wherein because of their self described "most highly evolved culture" whites are destined to rise to the top and rule the world, dominant over people of color.

[30] Adopt culture, behavior and grooming and as much as possible the appearance of white people.

[31] Marimba Ani, Yurugu. Asilli is "The logos of a culture, within which its various aspects cohere. It is the developmental germ/seed of a culture. It is the cultural essence, the ideological core, the matrix of a cultural entity which must be identified in order to make sense of the collective creations of its members."

[32] As immortalized in Two Thousand Seasons by Ayi Kwei Armah. AFDJ (2009).

[33] Wikipedia: Ori, literally meaning "head," refers to one's spiritual intuition and destiny. It is the reflective spark of human consciousness embedded into the human essence, and therefore is often personified as an Orisha in its own right. In Yoruba tradition, it is believed that human beings are able to heal themselves both spiritually and physically by working with the Orishas to achieve a balanced character, or *iwa-pele*. When one has a balanced character, one obtains an alignment with one's Ori or *divine self*.

Alignment with one's Ori brings, to the person who obtains it, inner peace and satisfaction with life. To come to know the Ori is, essentially, to come to know oneself, a concept extremely foreign to Western philosophy. The primacy of individual identity is best captured in a Yoruba proverb: "Ori la ba bo, a ba f'orisa sile". When translated, this becomes *It is the inner self we ought to venerate, and let divinity be.*

[34] In the Yoruba pantheon, Elegba is a deity, the divine messenger of Oludumare (God, the supreme being.) Elegba is a guardian, protector and communicator. Elegba is the Orisha that makes opportunities.

[35] Sankofa is a Twi term of the Akan of West Afrika. Sankofa is an Adinkra symbol and a concept represented graphically by a bird with his head turned around facing backwards. Sankofa is to move forward by looking backwards. The Sankofa process as written in The Sankofa Movement is the process of reafrikanization, the process of going back and claiming what culturally was ours in order to move forward as a people.

[36] Kobi K.K. Kambon, Cultural misorientation is the state of being in which a person functions culturally with a foreign mindset and cultural character.

[37] Laila Afrika, Nutricide (EWorld Inc. January 9, 2001). Nutritional suicide. Suicide by eating foods inappropriate for human consumption.

[38] Mesmerism is the sate of being transfixed and unaware of the reality of things around you.

[39] Karma is a Hindu/Buddhist term. According to dictionary.com: action, seen as bringing upon oneself inevitable results, good or bad, either in this life or in a reincarnation. *Theosophy* the cosmic principle according to which each person is rewarded or punished in one incarnation according to that person's deeds in the previous incarnation.

[40] John Stauber, *Mad Cow USA: The Nightmare Begins*, AlterNet, December 30, 2003.

[41] Michael Greger, *The Killer Among Us,* AlterNet, January 7, 2004.

[42] Michelle Alexander, The New Jim Crow (The New Press; January 5, 2010).

[43] God, the supreme being/entity. Yoruba.

[44] The drive resulting from one's asilli.

[45] Nananom (Akan), Egungun (Yoruba) = ancestors.

[46] Abossom (Akan), Orisha (Yoruba), Loa (Voudon) are deities manifesting a personified aspect of God.

[47] Cultural misorientation is the sate of thinking and behaving in a cultural framework that is foreign to the individual. Most specifically is refers to Afrikans thinking and behaving as if they were European. Kobi K.K, Kambon, Cultural Misorientation: The Greatest Threat To The Survival Of The Black Race In The 21st Century (Nubian Nation Publications 2003).

[48] Originally coined by Bobby E. Wright. According to Mwalimu Baruti, in <u>Mentacide</u> (Akoben House), mentacide occurs when you willingly think and act out of someone else's interpretation of reality to their benefit and against your survival. It is a state of subtle insanity which, over the last few hundred years, has come to characterize more and more Afrikans globally.

[49] Amos Wilson, <u>The Falsification Of Afrikan Consciousness</u> (1993 World InfoSystems).

[50] Joel Glodsmith, <u>Conscious Union with God</u> (Acropolis Books (GA); 1st Acropolis books edition June 2000).

[51] ibid.

100114-100-1-60W